Dr Marcia Wilkinson is Honorary Medical Director of the City of London Migraine Clinic and former Director of the Regional Neurological Unit at the Eastern Hospital, London. She was also Consultant Neurologist at the famous Elizabeth Garrett Anderson Hospital for women.

A migraine sufferer herself, she has had a lifelong active professional interest in the condition. She has written numerous articles on migraine and headaches, and has lectured on the subject around the world.

Dr Wilkinson lives in London. Her main leisure interests are gardening and walking.

MIGRAINE & HEADACHES

Understanding, controlling and
avoiding the pain

Dr Marcia Wilkinson
DM, FRCP

Medical Director
City of London Migraine Clinic

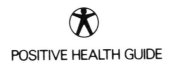

POSITIVE HEALTH GUIDE

To my daughters, Ottilie and Armine

© Dr Marcia Wilkinson 1982
Reprinted 1982
Reprinted 1984

First published in the United Kingdom in 1982
by Martin Dunitz Limited, London
This edition published in 1991 by
Macdonald Optima, a division of
Macdonald & Co. (Publishers) Ltd

A member of Maxwell Macmillan Pergamon Publishing Corporation

British Library Cataloguing in Publication Data
Wilkinson, Marcia
    Migraine and headaches.—rev. ed.
    1. Man. Head. Headaches
    I. Title II. Series
    616.8491

ISBN 0-356-19732-8

Macdonald & Co. (Publishers) Ltd
Orbit House
1 New Fetter Lane
London EC4A 1AR

CONTENTS

Introduction   6
1. What is migraine?   7
2. Who has migraine?   13
3. What are the symptoms?   19
4. Trigger factors   27
5. Women and migraine   41
6. What can you do to help yourself?   48
7. How can your doctor help?   56
8. Tension headache   64
9. Other headaches   69
10. Children and headaches   78
11. Research and migraine clinics   85
12. Stress and relaxation
(by Jane Madders, Dip P Ed, MCSP)   94
13. Conclusion   103
Useful addresses   104
Acknowledgements   106
Index   107

INTRODUCTION

Headache is one of the commonest complaints that afflicts mankind and one of the oldest. Some 30 per cent of the Western population suffer from headaches or, put another way, one in three people has one or more headaches a year.

There are probably over a hundred different types of headache but two of the commonest are migraine and tension headache, sometimes known as muscle contraction headache. Out of a hundred people coming to a migraine clinic with headache, about sixty-five will be suffering from migraine, about twenty-five from tension headache, and about ten from headaches due to other causes.

It is always difficult to get accurate statistics on the occurrence of headache for although most people have a headache at some time in their life, many never seek medical advice. Others have come to accept their headache as an inevitable part of their life and do not like to bother their doctor. In this book I will try to show what you can do to help yourself if you have a headache and offer some practical suggestions for coping with the stresses that may bring it on. Fortunately, most headaches are not a sign of serious disease, but if the pain is persistent and severe and the headaches are frequent then you should see your family doctor, who can then advise you on the best form of treatment for your particular type of headache. An understanding of the symptoms is often a help in coping with them and one of the first things most sufferers want to know is: what exactly is migraine? This is not simple to answer since the condition can assume different forms in different people; but in the opening chapters I shall explain what the various types of migraine are, and look at what sort of people suffer from them.

Please note
Although equivalent names are given in the book for drugs marketed in different countries, one product cannot be precisely equated with another due to variations in inactive substances which are added for coating and bulk.

1 WHAT IS MIGRAINE?

Migraine is a common ailment characterized by severe recurring headache. The headaches are usually on one side of the head, but may occasionally be on both sides. The pain varies greatly in severity, ranging from a dull nagging ache to an unbearable pounding. A number of other symptoms can accompany the headache: you may find that you have no appetite for food, or that you feel nauseous and are sick. Sometimes symptoms appear before the headache comes on and you may have trouble seeing or speaking, or you may feel giddy.

There is more than one kind of migraine and you may find that your attacks take different forms at different times. The three main types are: classical migraine, common migraine, and cluster headache or migrainous neuralgia. The International Headache Society has recently brought out a new classification. Classical migraine is called migraine with aura, and common migraine is now known as migraine without aura.

Classical migraine

With this type of migraine you will get a warning of an impending attack. Very often this takes the form of difficulties with your sight. Your vision may be blurred or you may have partial loss of sight. Sometimes there is a temporary inability to speak, and occasionally you may experience some disturbance in feeling and touch. Doctors call these warning symptoms the aura. They precede the headache and are thought to be caused by a narrowing of the blood vessels supplying a particular part of the brain.

Headache begins soon after the appearance of these symptoms and the pain is generally very severe. In two people out of three the headache is one-sided and usually recurs on the same side. But you may find that it occasionally occurs on the other side or on both sides at once.

Nausea and vomiting often accompany the headache and in a bad attack you will probably have to lie down. Diarrhoea is also associated with some migraine attacks.

Common migraine

As its name implies, common migraine is encountered more frequently. Unlike classical migraine, there are generally no warning symptoms or aura. However, the headache pain can be just as severe and cause equal distress. It is usually accompanied by nausea and vomiting. Occasionally you may feel nauseous before the headache comes on, and sometimes, after vomiting, there is some relief from the headache but sudden movements or bending down tend to make it worse. Between attacks of either classical or common migraine you will be free of all symptoms.

Cluster headache

Cluster headaches (migrainous neuralgia) – less usual than the classical or common forms of migraine – tend to occur in bouts or clusters which can last from two weeks to three months, with headache-free intervals between bouts lasting from a few months to three or four years. In bad attacks the headaches may occur several times in twenty-four hours, each headache pain lasting for anything up to two hours. Men are four times as likely as women to be affected by this type of migraine though doctors still do not fully understand why. Fortunately, only about 4 per cent of migraine sufferers get this particular kind of attack.

The pain is very intense and often located behind the eye. It may be accompanied by reddening and watering of the eye and by blockage of the nostril on the affected side.

You and your migraine

When did you first get it?

Migraine is essentially a disorder of the younger person. In fact, many people have their first attack in childhood. Any severe or persistent headache coming on for the first time after the age of fifty requires full investigation by your doctor. Pain which occurs every day, which is always there, and which is not made worse or better by anything, except perhaps stress, is usually due to tension (see chapter eight).

If you have had a long history of recurring headache and if the pain is sometimes on one side, sometimes on the other, the diagnosis of migraine is virtually certain. But it is important for anyone with sudden and severe headache to consult his or her doctor. People with headache are often worried that it may be an indication of something serious such as a brain tumour. Your family doctor will be able to take a complete history and give a full examination. The great majority of patients who go to their doctor complaining of headache, however, do not have any serious organic disease.

At what time of day do you get it?
Most migraine headaches start early in the morning, between 5 and 10 a.m. It is less usual for them to come on late in the day. Headaches caused by high blood pressure are present on waking, but tend to improve as soon as you get up and about. Cluster headaches can strike at any time and may even wake you during the night. Similarly, tension headaches can come on at any time of the day.

How long will it last?
The early warning symptoms in a classical migraine attack usually do not last more than fifteen to twenty minutes. The headache itself may last from an hour or two to about a day, or even two days. It is always advisable to take remedial action as early as possible in an attack (see chapter six). Sometimes, you can lessen the severity of the headache by acting as soon as you get the first indications that an attack is impending.

Migraine headaches can occur between one and eight times a month. Daily headaches, except the cluster headaches, are never due to migraine. Characteristically, the migraine headache does not come on when you are in hospital. If you are pregnant you are less likely to have an attack, and although much has been written about menstrual migraine, probably not more than 10 per cent of women with migraine have all or most of their headaches at the time of their period. We shall be looking at women and migraine more closely in chapter five.

Diagnosis

Diagnosis of a headache is a very complicated matter and one question I am often asked is: how is migraine different from other headaches? This is difficult to answer, particularly as it is possible for someone to suffer from more than one kind of headache. Before starting treatment for any kind of headache it is essential to make a diagnosis.

Is it eye trouble?

If the headache is felt behind the eye and comes on, or is made worse, when the eyes are moved or touched, the pain may be caused by some infection or trouble in the eye. An examination by your family doctor will confirm whether this is the case or not.

Have a dental check-up

Other common causes of pain in the head and face are tooth decay, impacted wisdom teeth, a malaliquid bite or other dental problems. Anyone with a constant dull ache in the face or head, particularly if it is accompanied by sharp jabs of pain, should have a dental check-up. This will normally include an X-ray which will enable your dentist to locate the source of the pain if it is caused by a troublesome tooth or abnormalities of the tempero-mandivular joint.

Neck ache

Some people develop pain in the back of the neck and head and occasionally this pain is associated with changes in the upper part of the cervical spine. Minor changes in the spine occur in most people over the age of fifty; generally they do not cause pain but there are some types of headache, particularly if the pain is in the back of the neck, which are associated with changes in the upper part of the cervical spine. If you do have pain in the back of your head or neck you should see your doctor.

What happens in a migraine attack

From earliest times people have tried to explain what causes migraine. In ancient Egyptian times and even later the symptoms were thought to be due to evil spirits and holes were sometimes made in the head (trephining) to let the evil spirits out. In the seventeenth century, after William Harvey had discovered that the blood circulates round the body, it was thought that migraine was primarily a disorder of the blood vessels. The present view is that migraine is probably due to biochemical changes in the brain and that the changes in the blood vessels are secondary to this. But there is still a lot of discussion about why this happens as different things seem to trigger off attacks in different people.

The mechanisms of migraine

While there is no doubt that changes in the size of the blood vessels take place during a migraine attack, it is still not fully understood how or why. However, it seems most likely that the changes in the blood vessels are secondary to the increased production of one or more of the following biochemical substances in the body:

Catecholamines   These are hormones produced by the adrenal glands and include adrenalin, noradrenalin and dopamine. These are among the substances released in the body when you are under stress. Research workers have suggested that there may be a difference in the controlling mechanism for the production, breakdown and storage of these substances in people with migraine.

Histamine   This is a substance produced by the body in response to injury shock or during an allergic reaction. It can cause the blood vessels either to contract or dilate. At one time

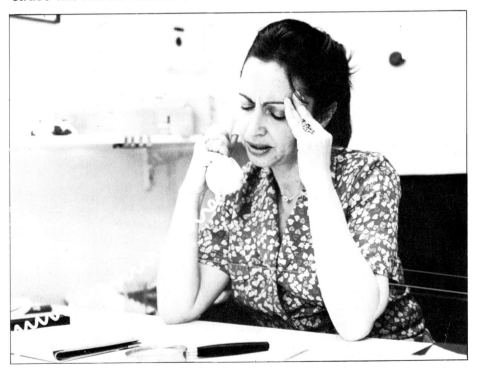

This sort of stressful situation releases hormones such as adrenalin, and in susceptible people this can result in a migraine attack.

migraine sufferers were thought to be particularly sensitive to histamine, but headaches induced by injections of histamine are not now thought to be like migraine headaches.

Serotonin   This is a chemical which is found in the brain and is released from tissues in the body into the bloodstream. Serotonin can influence the size of the blood vessels throughout the body. Research has shown that during migraine attacks there are changes in the blood serotonin (see page 88).

Prostaglandins   These are chemicals in the body known to be closely involved in the production of pain. They also have considerable effect on the blood vessels.

One of the difficulties in finding out what happens during a migraine attack is that substances which may be involved in an attack are only produced just before the attack or in the very early stages, and unless samples of blood or urine are taken from the sufferer at this time no abnormalities will be found. This is one of the reasons why a clinic such as the City of London Migraine Clinic, with which I have been associated for many years, is important, because here people can be seen early in an attack and research into these changes in the body can be done.

All kinds of people come to the City of London Migraine Clinic for advice and help, but as most people with headaches do not go to their doctor at all, we must look beyond clinics to find out more about who has migraine.

2 WHO HAS MIGRAINE?

How common is migraine?

It is probable that at least one in ten people suffer from migraine and that about one in three have some kind of headache in the course of a year. In a recent survey it was found that only 20 per cent of those who had migraine in the previous year had seen a doctor because of their headaches, and that about half had never consulted a doctor about their headaches at any time. Again, in a later similar study it was found that only one in two hundred people who complained of headaches had actually consulted their doctor, while a house-to-house survey showed that many more had had headaches at some time in the previous year, in fact, six times as many as had asked for advice.

The cost of migraine

If one in ten people have migraine that means that in a country such as Britain over 6 million people will suffer from it – about 1½ million men and 4½ million women. If about half these people are working and each loses one day from work each twelve months, that represents a loss to the nation's output of 3 million working days per year. Migraine, therefore, is not only a great burden for the sufferer but also a drain on a nation's resources.

Although it is often considered to be a minor disorder by those who have never suffered from it, when the cost of migraine is added up, it is of considerable economic importance. When the amount paid for drugs is added to the cost of the days lost, the bill becomes enormous. In the United States alone more than $500 million is spent annually on medication by those seeking relief from headache. Most migraine sufferers have at least four headaches a year and if two pills of aspirin or paracetamol (Acetaminophen in the United States) are taken for each headache – which is probably a great deal less than the number actually used – you can see that migraine is an expensive business.

Are migraine sufferers above average intelligence?

It has been said that migraine mainly affects those in professional or managerial occupations; there is, however, no evidence that this is true. What is true is that of those who ask their doctors for advice a higher proportion come from the professional and managerial classes. Some of the original research on the number of headaches and the occupations of those who get them was done by a group of New York physicians with large private practices in the city, and their figures reflect the kind of patients you would expect to find attending these kinds of medical practices. Other, recent studies have shown that migraine affects all groups of the population.

The table below shows the results of an analysis of the occupations of two thousand patients attending the City of London Migraine Clinic:

Occupation	Number seen	Percentage
Administrative and clerical	640	32.0
Housewife	452	22.6
Executive and professional	299	15.0
Skilled	198	9.9
Student	134	6.7
Manual	114	5.7
Other	124	6.2
Unknown	39	1.9
	2,000	100.0

These figures may at first seem to support the idea that more intelligent people get migraine, but in fact the high percentage of those doing administrative or clerical work, or who are of professional or executive status, merely reflects the fact that the clinic is in the City of London where the majority of people work in offices, and there are relatively few manual workers. Although there are only a few housewives in the City, they have time during the day to come in to the Clinic from the suburbs.

Nevertheless, there are a number of famous intelligent people who have had migraine. One of the most renowned was Charles Lutwidge Dodgson, a mathematician and writer of nonsense, better known as Lewis Carroll, the author of *Alice's Adventures in Wonderland* (1865). Many of the things that happened in the book to Alice can be explained on a migrainous basis: for instance, the Cheshire cat who appears and disappears, or sometimes is only partly visible. This is the sort of visual trick which can happen in a migraine attack when perhaps the left-hand side of something can be seen but not the right. In an attack objects may seem bigger or smaller than usual. This could have given Lewis Carroll the idea for the bottle with 'drink me' on it which made Alice smaller and for the cake with 'eat me' on it which made her bigger.

Other famous people who suffered from migraine include Calvin, Queen Mary Tudor, the first Duke of Marlborough, the philosophers Pascal and Nietzsche, and Sigmund Freud. Thomas Jefferson had terrible headaches for much of his life as did Ulysses S. Grant.

Does migraine affect more women than men?

The list of famous people with migraine is misleading in one respect because it contains more men than women. In fact, the number of women with migraine exceeds the number of men with migraine by about three to one.

One of the questions I am often asked is: why is this so? The most likely answer is that in women there is a constant change in the hormonal pattern during the menstrual cycle, and this may be one of the things that causes headaches. Many women, but not all, find that their migraine is better when they are pregnant and often migraine improves after the change of life.

Surprisingly perhaps, among young children boys have migraine slightly more often than girls. After puberty the number of girls with migraine catches up with the number of boys and by the age of twenty more women than men have migraine.

Is age a factor?

Many people get their first migraine headache as a child; it comes on early in life – even a two-year-old can suffer from it – and is primarily a disorder of the under-fifties. The average age of those attending a migraine clinic is thirty-eight. The graph given here shows the age at the time of the first headache attack in some 1,800 people:

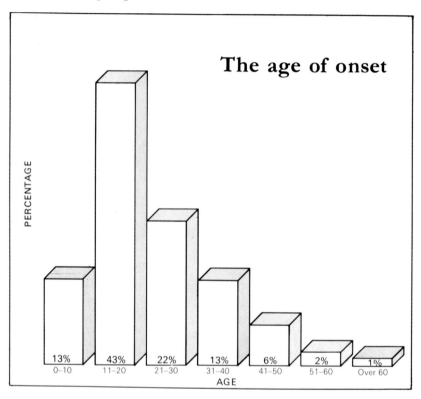

This graph shows at what age the first migraine attack is likely to occur. The vast majority of sufferers have theirs before the age of forty.

The figures show that more than half the people in the survey had their first headache before the age of twenty and that over 90 per cent had had a migraine attack before they were forty. It is rare to develop migraine over the age of fifty and if you do begin to get headaches at this age the cause is probably not migraine.

In most people migraine attacks tend to get fewer after the age of forty-five. The reason for this is not known for certain;

but there is, perhaps, less variation in the hormonal pattern after the age of fifty.

Is migraine inherited?

Many people want to know whether they are more likely to get migraine if there is already someone in their family with it. Some are also worried that they might pass it on to their children. But whatever is inherited, it is certainly not the headache; either it is some biochemical abnormality, or an abnormality of one of the constituents of the blood, probably the platelets, or some type of psychological response to various environmental influences. In a family it may be very difficult to identify the latter.

There are many families in which more than one member suffers from migraine and it is likely that if you have migraine your father or mother may have had the same problem or your children will develop it. All doctors know of such families and if you go to see your doctor about your migraine, one of the questions he will probably ask you is do any of the rest of the family have headaches? The answer is likely to be yes in over 60 per cent of cases, especially if grandmothers, aunts and uncles are included. At least one in ten of the population has migraine and therefore statistically every extended family of ten people or more should have at least one sufferer.

The predisposition to headache – rather than the headache itself – is inherited, and in anyone the headaches may be triggered off by any number of things – foods, fasting, lack of sleep, or stress. The following is a typical case history.

Pamela Watson, aged forty, came to see me on account of her severe headaches. She said that her mother had told her that her grandmother had suffered from sick headaches when she was a young woman. Pamela had two daughters aged fourteen and seven. The elder daughter developed headaches at the age of twelve when she moved from the junior to the senior school. These were at first thought to be tension headaches, but in the last year she had developed classical migraine, with visual disturbances, nausea and vomiting. Her seven-year-old daughter did not have headaches but was often travel sick. Pamela had herself been car-sick as a child and had started her headaches when she was studying at university. She had continued to have headaches, together with nausea and vomiting, since then. They usually came on when she was worried or upset. The diagnosis of migraine was confirmed after examination and some anti-sickness pills and a pain-killer were prescribed. Her headaches gradually improved.

Travel sickness

It is interesting that Pamela and her younger daughter both suffered from travel sickness at some time. Many people with migraine have a history of having been travel sick as a child. This may be not only sea-sickness, but also sickness in a car or a bus. If you are travelling with a child prone to travel sickness, it is best to go prepared with bucket and tissues. Often children are less likely to be sick if they sit in the front seat or in a position where they can see what is going on. Travel sickness will often lessen as the child gets older.

3 WHAT ARE THE SYMPTOMS?

The three main symptoms in migraine are, as we have seen, headache, nausea and vomiting, and – in classical migraine – the visual symptoms which precede the attack, the aura. We shall be looking at these in greater detail in this chapter but it is perhaps a good idea to point out here that migraine is an episodic disturbance. This means that it comes and goes at intervals; between attacks you will feel quite normal and the fact that you suffer at times from migraine should not prevent you from leading a perfectly normal life for the rest of the time.

Early signs

You may be one of the many sufferers who know the previous day that they are going to have a migraine attack. You may have a feeling of heaviness of the head, or be aware of slight discomfort or pain, feel sleepy or yawn. Sometimes you feel abnormally well before an attack and may wish to go out for a meal or do some vigorous spring-cleaning. But when an attack consists of a headache only, characteristically you will wake up with it.

Before the attack – the aura

In classical migraine, before the attack comes on, you may experience some unusual sensations called the aura. These sensations are different for everyone who has them and they are usually, but not always, visual. They may consist of flashing or zigzagging lights, dimness of vision, a sensation of looking through water, or even blindness in one part of the visual field. Very often the difficulty in seeing is limited to one side, so you find you cannot see well on the right side with the right eye, or on the right side with your left eye (or vice versa). Medically this is known as hemianopia; and although it can, of course, be a very frightening experience, it is not uncommon among those who suffer from classical migraine. Fortunately, these difficulties in vision do not last very long, generally between fifteen and forty minutes. Most people like to lie down in a quiet darkened room when they have this kind of disturbance.

A bright spot may appear

You may feel perfectly well but suddenly be conscious of a bright spot on one side of your vision. This may slowly enlarge and spread, becoming darker in the centre as it extends, and changing its round outline into an angular form. A detailed description of the visual disturbances that can occur in a migraine attack was given in the late nineteenth century by a physician writing a text book on diseases of the nervous system, Dr William Gowers.

He describes a series of strange spectral appearances, some of which you may be familiar with through your own experience of these phenomena.

> Very commonly the outer edge of the bright spot assumes a zigzag shape with prominent and re-entrant angles, like the ground plan of a fortification, and hence called 'fortification spectrum'. At one part it becomes fainter and ceases so that there is a break in the outline. The outer boundary is the most brilliant and is often limited by colours; inside the luminosity extends for a little distance gradually becoming fainter. Very frequently within the bright outline, sparks arise. There seem to be numerous particles in rapid regular movement. The spectrum increases with the blind area, gradually becomes indistinct, and disappears at the periphery of the field.

Sometimes the visual disturbances are not followed by headache. In fact, it is not unusual for some changes in the nature of your migraine to occur at certain periods as the following case history shows:

Kelly Atkinson, now aged fifty, had one-sided headaches as a child which were often associated with sickness. On one occasion, when she was about fourteen, she was taken out shopping by her mother – an activity which she did not enjoy. They went from shop to shop looking for a suitable coat which they were unable to find. Her mother was in a hurry because she had booked seats for the cinema, and so took a taxi. By this time Kelly was feeling anxious as well as nauseated and had a bad headache. When her mother exclaimed: 'Look at that procession of soldiers on horseback!' Kelly put her head out of the window to see the procession and was promptly sick.

Her headaches continued after this, usually coming on at times of stress, often with a feeling of sickness and occasionally vomiting. During her twenties the headaches became less troublesome and she was free of headaches when she was having her children.

In her late thirties the symptoms changed again and she tended to get visual disturbances without any headache. The disturbances of vision were usually on the left side and consisted of ovals of scintillating jagged light which formed and reformed. Each time she tried to look at them they went away, only to come back almost immediately. In addition to the lights there was a shimmering, floating appearance in front of her eyes and she was unable to read. These symptoms passed off in about fifteen minutes.

The first time that these occurred, Kelly was very alarmed and upset as she was convinced that they were due to some serious brain condition but as they recurred, she began to accept them, knowing that they would go in under half-an-hour. She was advised by her doctor to rest if she could during an attack and take her tablets. She still has the occasional attack but is now able to take the appropriate treatment early in the attack and thus minimize its severity.

A tingling feeling
Sometimes you may get a tingling feeling or numbness in one side of the face or round the lips, or else have pins and needles down one side of your body. Occasionally, there may be a weakness in one of your arms or legs, lasting up to ten or fifteen minutes. Or the tingling may begin in one hand and slowly spread up the arm. As it subsides the headache comes on.

Difficulty in speaking
A less common warning symptom of an attack is speech disturbance and mental confusion. Again it is a worrying symptom, especially if you find you are unable to say the right word or express what you mean, but it passes off and generally only lasts a few minutes.

Trouble with hearing and balance

About half of those suffering from migraine may experience some distortion of sounds or other hearing difficulty, as well as a sensation of giddiness. Dislike of noise is quite common, but sometimes you may be aware of mumbles and hisses or suffer a partial loss of hearing. Even your own voice may take on an unreal quality. Elizabeth Garrett Anderson, an English physician and pioneer in the professional education of women, wrote a thesis on migraine in 1870 in which she says: 'the patient dreads noise, light or the slightest movement and is tormented by the vibration of a pendulum.' Any loud noise, she wrote, may make the headache worse.

Loss of balance or giddiness occur fairly often. You may feel that your surroundings are spinning round you. As with the hearing difficulties, giddiness may either precede or accompany the headache.

Headache

This is the symptom most people associate with migraine. It can vary in severity from a mild but bearable ache to an incapacitating throbbing pain which leaves the sufferer exhausted. Super-imposed on the throbbing pain, which has also been likened to a series of hammer blows, there may be a sharp jabbing pain, like being stabbed in the head with a nail or needle. If untreated, the headache may last for hours, even days, but if you can lie down and take a pain-killer, or whatever drug your doctor has recommended, the pain generally eases after one or two hours.

Variation on a theme

The site of the headache may vary from attack to attack. Dr J. Oleson of Copenhagen investigated 678 patients with migraine and found six distinct areas where headache pain was felt:

Areas of pain	Percentage
One-sided headache	44
Pain all over the head	22
Pain at the front of the head (on both sides)	14
Frontal one-sided pain	13
Back of the head	6
Crown of the head (vertex)	1

Sometimes people have classical migraine as children but as they get older the visual disturbances may cease, and they get only the headache. In other cases, where they have had headache alone, sensory disturbances may occur later. One of my patients at the City of London Migraine Clinic had loss of vision on one side with his migraine attacks until he was about fifty. The visual symptom then stopped, but he went on having headaches. Another patient who had a strong family history of migraine had had simple, sick headaches – that is, headaches associated with nausea and vomiting – since he was a child. At twenty-five he had slight concussion after a fall in which he hit his head against a wall. He subsequently experienced loss of vision on one side followed by headache, and from that time on each migraine attack was preceded by this visual disorder.

Nausea and vomiting

Nausea and vomiting occur at some time in the majority of those with migraine. Sometimes the feeling is that of unwillingness to eat and a general distaste for food. At other times there is vomiting and this may be one of the most distressing features of the attack. It also makes treatment difficult because if someone is nauseated or vomiting, the pills taken by mouth are unlikely to have much effect. They may be vomited back and there is evidence that drugs taken by mouth in a migraine attack may not be absorbed properly.

Some very interesting recent work has shown that while patients with migraine absorbed aspirin normally when they were headache free, in a migraine attack the absorption of aspirin was definitely slower and less complete. Another interesting finding was that if a drug called metoclopramide was given to people suffering from migraine, their absorption of aspirin during an attack became virtually normal. It is difficult to measure the actual activity of the stomach itself, but it is relatively easy to see whether the stomach is absorbing such substances as aspirin or alcohol at the same rate under different conditions.

In addition to nausea and vomiting, about one in five sufferers may also have disturbance of their bowel movements and diarrhoea may occur. This happens only during the attack and bowel action is normal between attacks. Failure to pass water during the early part of a migraine attack is quite common and nothing to worry about. As the migraine gets better you may notice that you pass water more frequently than usual; this too is no cause for alarm.

What else might you feel?

Most people in a migraine attack look pale and feel cold and if you are one of these sufferers, it is as well to go to bed with a hot-water bottle and, if you are not feeling too sick, to have a cup of hot sweet tea. On the other hand some people feel hot and their faces are flushed during an attack.

Scalp tenderness
This may occur during or after an attack in about half of those with migraine. Sometimes it is merely an unpleasant sensation when you comb or brush your hair, or it may be severe enough to stop you lying down on the affected side. This feeling of tenderness can involve any part of the head or neck.

Water retention
This can come on hours or days before the actual migraine attack. It is quite common to find that you have put on 2 or 3 lb (1 or 1½ kg) in weight at this time and some people find that their rings or clothes feel tight. Very often these people pass a lot of urine either at the peak of the headache or as it gradually gets better. Drugs known as diuretics (which help you to pass water) have been tried, but they do not usually prevent the migraine attack.

Nasal stuffiness
Somewhere between 10 and 20 per cent of migraine sufferers complain of nasal stuffiness. The symptoms tend to last until the headache goes.

Fever
Children sometimes have a fever with migraine and their temperatures may rise alarmingly. Temperatures as high as 40°C (104°F) have been reported. If you are in any doubt about your child it is best to get in touch with your doctor.

Rapid heartbeat
This has been found in about 3 per cent of migraine attacks. It nearly always improves as the headache wears off.

Changes in mood
Slight mood changes occur in some people before or during an attack. You may find that you feel depressed and restless, or even that you are slightly confused. Sometimes there is a temporary loss of memory. Some people feel that they are 'not really there' soon after the beginning of an attack. This may well happen when the attack is preceded by unusual sensory disturbances. Among other unusual sensations that have been described to me by patients is a feeling of 'double consciousness' or vivid recollection of events long past.

Rare forms of migraine

There is a very rare type of migraine called hemiplegic migraine in which there is a recurrent weakness of one side of the body. Very often there is a history of a similar kind of attack in the family and usually the weakness is on the same side in both mother and daughter, or, less often, father and son. The treatment for this is the same as for classical migraine but before hemiplegic migraine is diagnosed, all other possible causes for a weakness on one side of the body must be excluded. Anybody with this symptom should go and see his or her doctor who will probably arrange for an examination by a neurologist. This will possibly include something called a CAT scan (the letters stand for computerized axial tomography) which is a complicated but quite painless type of X-ray.

Another uncommon type is ophthalmoplegic migraine, in which there is weakness in one or more of the muscles that move the eye or some abnormality of the pupil. Again, anyone who has this condition should go and see their family doctor and all other possible causes should be excluded before a diagnosis of migraine is made.

The term 'migraine equivalent' is used to describe the migraine symptoms which occur without a headache or with only a very mild one. The diagnosis of a migraine equivalent can only be made if the symptoms occur as regularly, and last as long, as the migraine attack, and are triggered off by similar factors. Just what is most likely to bring on a migraine is a subject I shall examine in the next chapter.

4 TRIGGER FACTORS

Ask any group of people with migraine what brings on their attacks and you will get a wide variety of answers. Nevertheless, there are a number of things which seem to be on virtually everyone's list. They are:

Changes in daily routine
Sleep – too much or too little
Excitement
Noise
Light
Certain foods (a great number have been blamed)
Stress
Effort and exercise
The weather
Smells
Hormonal factors

If you have migraine you should try to find out what your own particular trigger factors are. Keep a careful diary listing the migraine attacks, monthly periods and anything that might have precipitated the attacks. You may find the above list helpful in pinpointing what brings them on. We shall be looking at each of the factors in turn.

Changes in daily routine

Any change in routine, such as a new job, shift work, vacations – all of which can give rise to a feeling of uncertainty – can set off an attack of migraine. It doesn't even have to be a disagreeable change. Indeed, some people find that their headaches are worse at the weekend.

Weekend headache
There are two possible explanations for weekend headache.

One is that after a hard week's work the Saturday headache is a 'release' headache which comes on when the pressure of work is relieved.

The other explanation is that the weekend is often a time of stress, particularly for the working mother, as it is then she has to cope with her family and all the household problems. Studies show, however, that objectively speaking there is no significant difference between the various days of the week. If you find that the weekend is a bad time for you, try getting the rest of the family to help with some of the chores. For some, an extra hour or two in bed is the answer, but occasionally too much sleep can bring on a headache.

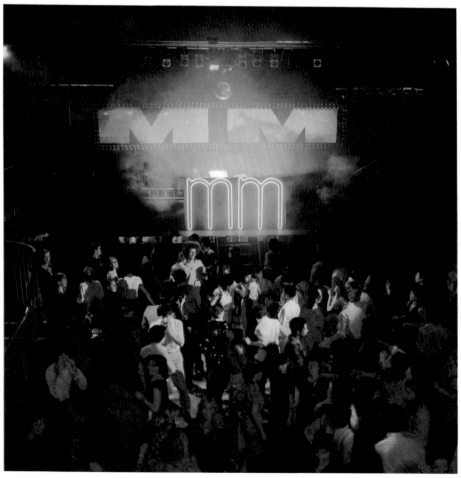

Disco dancing is not a recommended activity for those prone to migraine. Excitement, flashing lights and loud music can all trigger off an attack.

Sleep

Although most people find that they feel better if they can lie down and go to sleep when they have a migraine attack, a few find that if they sleep very late in the morning they have a headache when they wake up. If this is the case with you, it is best to stick to regular hours and get to bed at about the same time each night and rise at the same time each morning.

On the other hand, you may get a headache if you haven't had enough sleep. Staying up late, or being unable to sleep at night, does seem to bring on an attack in certain people.

Excitement

Another common trigger factor is excitement. This is particularly noticeable in children (see chapter ten), but even adults can feel the effects of an evening out and the result may be a headache the next morning. Some social occasions can be stressful, especially for shy people, but very often it is a combination of factors which brings on the headache. For example, not only do most people tend to drink more at social gatherings, but they may also feel anxious at the thought of meeting new people; the food may be different from what they usually eat and there may also be extra noise and, sometimes, uncomfortably bright lighting.

Noise and light

Many people find that glaring lights or loud noises are liable to give them headaches, but those with migraine are particularly susceptible. When asked, they usually say that the noise has to be loud and persistent or the light unbearable. Their one wish in these circumstances is to find somewhere quiet and dark to lie down so that they can relax and go to sleep.

This wish for darkness and tranquillity has been used in the treatment room at the City of London Migraine Clinic. There, people are able to lie down and, having received the appropriate treatment, go to sleep if they want to. My experience has shown me that patients are much more likely to get over a migraine quickly if they are able to go to sleep in a quiet dark room, so in the Clinic the shutters are drawn, the floor is carpeted and the beds are comfortable.

I first met Victor Zoppa when he was twenty-five. He had come to the Clinic complaining of headaches and said that he had had them since the age of eight. When they first started they came on only two or three times a year, often when he was excited at the thought of an outing – going to the circus, for example. Very often he was sick as well, but if he took an aspirin and was able to lie down the headache went away. After he left school he had no headaches for two or three years, but they had started again two years ago. They were now more severe and came on about once every six weeks. Before the headaches he experienced flashing lights on the right side – these lasted for about fifteen minutes – and then he developed a terrible pain over his left eye and felt sick. Unless he took some kind of pain-killer the pain lasted all day and he usually vomited after a few hours.

After talking with Victor I found that about two years ago he had decided to train as a computer clerk and part of his job involved watching continually changing numbers on a visual display unit (VDU) screen – similar to a television's. It was around this time that his headaches became significantly worse.

Victor eventually found another job and his headaches have since improved, though he is not completely free of them.

Light, particularly a flickering or glaring light, is often the cause of headache. Intermittent flashes, such as occur with poor fluorescent lighting or a badly adjusted television set can also trigger one off, so do adjust your television if it begins to play up.

Like Victor, a number of people working with computers have found that flickering screens can be a problem and it is very important to make sure that all electrical equipment is functioning properly.

Food

Is there a migraine diet?
For many years people have thought there might be a dietary cause for migraine and there is no doubt that during a migraine

attack most people have a distaste for food. Many feel nauseated and are sick, but this is probably because of the inactivity of the stomach during a migraine attack and is not primarily due to something they have eaten.

There is, though, good evidence that some people do find that certain foods bring on an attack. The ones most commonly blamed are alcohol, cheese and other dairy products, all forms of fried food, chocolate, citrus fruits, tea and coffee, and seafoods. Since these are a very common part of a normal diet it is difficult to know whether any one of these foods and drinks does bring on an attack.

It is of little use to go on a so-called migraine diet and exclude all the foods which have been accused of triggering an attack, because this could result in an unbalanced diet and lead you no nearer to discovering the food which most affects you. To find out whether a particular food triggers off an attack, the best thing for you to do is to exclude one food only from your diet for a period of a month and then see whether your headaches are significantly better. This can then be repeated with each of the other foods and drinks (see page 49).

What factors in food might cause migraine?

Dr Edda Hanington selected a group of patients who were attending the migraine clinic at the Elizabeth Garrett Anderson Hospital in London and had a clear-cut history of an association between certain types of food and their headaches. These patients were asked whether they would be willing to take part in an investigation. A trial was done where they were given either capsules containing 100 mg of tyramine – a chemical found in the body and also contained in certain foods – or similar capsules containing a placebo – a harmless, non-active substance – in this case lactose. She found that out of the sixty-six patients to whom she gave lactose, only six developed an attack within twenty-four hours, while among the hundred who had tyramine, eighty developed an attack. All the patients had previously been told not to take the capsules if they had had a headache in the previous forty-eight hours.

Tyramine is found mostly in substances which have undergone some bacterial decomposition such as certain cheeses and game, but the amount of tyramine present is not constant in any particular cheese and the amount in Cheddar may vary from a small amount to 100 mg in 4 oz (100 g). The cheeses in which

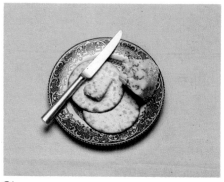

Cheese

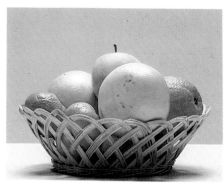

Citrus fruits

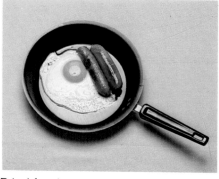

Fried food

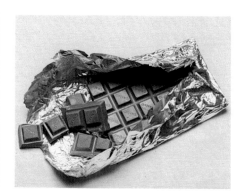

Chocolate

There is no doubt that certain foods can bring on migraine in some people. Illustrated on these two pages are those most frequently blamed. Chocolate is probably the worst offender, and least essential for a healthy diet.

the highest concentration has been found are Cheddar, Stilton and blue cheese. Tyramine belongs to a group of chemical compounds found in the body called amines, some of which play an important part in the working of the brain and in the circulation of the blood. They are also found in certain foods (as we have seen with tyramine). Another amine, octopamine, is present in citrus fruits, and dopamine is present in broad beans. Some people have noticed that their headaches come on after eating these foods.

Obviously, if you know a certain food or drink sets off an attack it is only wise to eliminate it from your diet. Some people have reported improvement after excluding bread, milk, tea, coffee or sugar; others have suggested that the real cause of the headache is an allergy or hypersensitivity to particular foods.

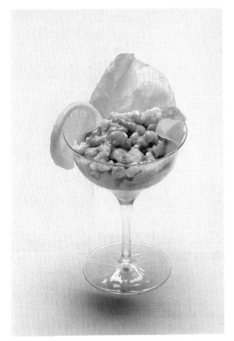
Sea-food

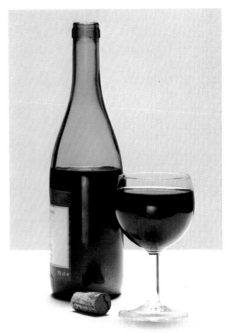
Red wine

Are you allergic to certain foods?

Allergy is a word with which most people are familiar. It can be defined as an unusual or exaggerated reaction to a substance or substances. In an allergic reaction there is usually swelling, inflammation and destruction of tissue. Any substance which causes the body to react in this particular way is called an allergen and an allergen may be almost anything from pollen to a bee sting or something that you eat. Migraine has sometimes been included among the allergic disorders and this was mainly because, like asthma and hay fever, the attack can be very severe and comes on at intervals.

Certain foods could precipitate a migraine attack either because they contain substances which act as allergens or because they contain chemically active constituents, such as tyramine or sodium nitrite, which may bring on headache. For instance, coffee taken in excess can cause headache because of the caffeine and other substances it contains.

One of the main difficulties in deciding whether a migraine patient has a food allergy or not is the lack of a clear-cut diagnostic test which will enable the doctor to say to which

33

particular food the patient is allergic. Advances in knowledge and technique have been made over the years and tests are now available, but these are difficult and expensive, and much more work needs to be done on them in controlled trials before they can be routinely applied.

Beware of rich, spicy food
John Fothergill writing over two hundred years ago expressed very succinctly what still holds true for migraine sufferers today:

> There are some things which in very small quantities seldom fail to produce a sick headache in some constitutions, such as a larger proportion than usual of melted butter, fat meat, spices, especially black pepper. Meat pies often contain all these things united and are as fertile a cause of this complaint as anything I know; rich baked puddings, and everything of a similar nature. A little error in these things will seldom fail to be attended with much suffering, in every constitution. Indeed, as the disorder comes on, mostly towards morning, the generality of patients are led to consider it as a thing impossible, that they should suffer so long after a meal; it is nevertheless true and ought to be strictly enquired into, and the conduct of the sick regulated in this respect, or medicine is exhibited in vain.

Cut down on chocolate
Chocolate is probably the commonest food with which people associate migraine attacks and in any survey over 60 per cent of people will probably mention this as a trigger factor. Chocolate has a complicated chemical structure and contains many different amines. Dr Hanington found that migraine attacks could be brought on in some patients by giving them one of the amines found in chocolate.

Chocolate is a relatively easy thing to exclude from your diet and you may find that you are better without it. There is always the added advantage that a diet free of chocolate will help you keep slim!

White wine rather than red
The hangover headache which comes on after drinking too much alcohol is well known and is probably due to the widening

of the blood vessels which occurs when too much is drunk. Even in small quantities alcohol causes a feeling of warmth and flushing of the face, and many alcoholic drinks also contain various amines such as tyramine, histamine and betaphenylethylamine. Red wine which has more amines in it than white, is particularly likely to bring on an attack and some sufferers prefer to enjoy a trouble-free glass of white wine.

During a bout of cluster headache even small amounts of alcohol will probably bring on an attack, although between the attacks most people are able to drink alcohol in reasonable quantities.

Stress

Mental or physical stress of any kind may trigger an attack of migraine. In fact, anyone who is tense or anxious or who has had an emotional shock is liable to develop a headache. We shall be looking at the headaches caused by tension in chapter eight but the advice to anyone who is under stress is the same: try to relax.

Even pleasant things can cause stress, such as promotion at work or going on vacation. Take, for example, the mother who is preparing for the family vacation. Not only does she have to see that all the packing has been done and that all her family is ready for the journey, but she has probably had to get up very early to prepare their breakfast, having not slept very well the previous night. Later in the day when they have been travelling in the car for several hours, one of the children may be car-sick and the car is probably hot and uncomfortable. In addition, she may not have had a proper lunch – just sausages, egg and chips at the roadside diner. When she gets to her destination she is tired out and finds that she can no longer cope with the family and she is by then suffering from a severe headache.

People with classical migraine are particularly susceptible to attacks triggered off by strong emotions. As one of the earliest authorities on migraine, Dr Liveing, wrote in 1870: 'It does not seem to matter much what the character of the emotion is provided it is strongly felt.'

Kenneth Naughton is a successful businessman who reached the top of his profession at the early age of thirty. He had occasional headaches as a child and these always came on when he was under stress. He did very well at school, winning a place in the football team as well as getting into university. In his late teens and early twenties he was relatively free of headaches and he soon got promotion in his firm. His present job involves long hours of work, heavy financial responsibilities and many crucial meetings.

His wife began to notice that he was getting increasingly irritable and that his headaches were becoming more frequent. These headaches were particularly likely to come on if he was upset, and she and the children dreaded going out in the car with him as any traffic hold-up made him furiously angry. After such an episode he would complain of feeling sick and of a throbbing left-sided headache which was so severe that he had to go to bed. Later he often vomited. His headaches improved when he was reassured at the Clinic and prescribed an anti-sickness drug and a pain-killer.

Stress is an unavoidable part of most people's lives today and we have to find ways of coping with it. For some people keeping fit is the answer. But make sure that you do not take up an exercise programme beyond your capabilities.

Effort and exercise

Lifting heavy weights, bending down and over-exertion are commonly cited as trigger factors. Certainly they are all things to avoid during an attack as they tend to make the headache worse. For a few people any type of physical exertion brings on a headache, usually at the back of the head and neck, and further effort makes the pain worse. Support of the neck muscles may help in this case as the underlying trouble could be in the cervical spine.

Are you fit?
Headache may also occur if you are unfit and suddenly start a series of strenuous exercises. The headache pain is intense and throbbing and often associated with a feeling of sickness. As your fitness improves, this type of headache should disappear. It is always wise to start any form of exercise gently, whether you are going jogging, playing tennis or squash, or just exercising at home.

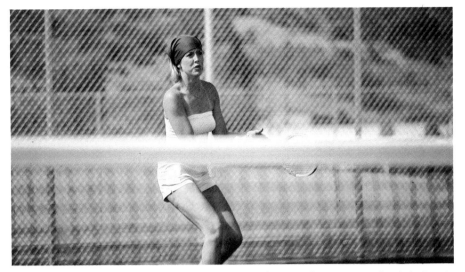

Over-exertion is a common migraine trigger factor. If you are unfit and plan to start playing tennis or take up some other sporting activity, take it easy at first.

Headaches and sport

Migraine may be brought on by the effort, both physical and mental, required in playing competitive games, or indeed by any kind of competitive activity.

Many athletes taking part in the 1968 Mexico City Olympic Games experienced acute one-sided headaches as well as feelings of nausea. This was probably mainly due to the intense exertion and excitement of the competition – effort migraine – but the symptoms were made worse by the altitude of 7,000 ft (2,100 m). Immediately after an event some athletes were conscious of visual disturbances – including temporary loss of sight – and a few minutes later they developed nausea and a severe throbbing headache behind the eye. A few unfortunate individuals had attacks after each heat, but the majority had only minor symptoms. In fit, well-trained athletes these symptoms rarely last long.

Even if you are not in training for the next Olympics you may find that a tense competitive game brings on an attack and it may be best for you to avoid such games. You could always try jogging like one of my patients.

Bob Dunsdale is an athletic man aged twenty-eight. He came to me with a history of childhood migraine. As a boy he had experienced visual disturbances consisting of bright zigzag lines which lasted between fifteen and twenty minutes. As he grew older the zigzag lines lasted longer. They were nearly always followed by a severe headache. He found that lying down made him feel worse and did not shorten his attack. He preferred to sit up and try to focus his eyes on some distant object. This seemed to make the zigzag effect more tolerable.

The unusual part of his story was that although he sometimes experienced the zigzag lines when playing football, he did not then develop a headache. He now goes jogging to ward off a headache.

One thing you cannot do much about is changes in the weather, which are frequently implicated in migraine attacks.

Migraine and the weather

Many people say that they know when a storm is coming because they feel irritable, depressed and cannot sleep. Some blame the heat or cold for their migraine attacks. Others say that a hot dry atmosphere is a cause of headache.

Generally speaking, however, it seems that headaches are more likely to be a result of the stress caused by unfavourable weather conditions rather than by the weather itself. For example, you may get a headache after a heavy snowfall when perhaps you have had to dig your car out or clear a path from your front door. In other words, several factors are operating in addition to the weather: physical effort in shovelling the snow, exposure to the cold, and anxiety about getting to work or the children off to school.

Many migraine sufferers do think that their headaches are brought on by the weather. Because of this some three hundred patients who attended a London migraine clinic were studied to see if atmospheric conditions could in any way be linked with their headaches.

The start of each attack was correlated with the direction and speed of the wind, and with the barometric pressure, temperature and humidity. For this group there did not appear to be any connection between the number and severity of attacks and adverse weather conditions. You must, of course, bear in mind that in the London area there are no great or sudden changes in the weather.

Another study showed that in Britain there is no one season which is 'better' or less stressful than the others. In the two years studied there were only three significant drops in the number of people attending the clinic: two in December – which probably represented the time taken for shopping and the Christmas vacation – and the other in June 1977 – the time of the Queen's Silver Jubilee celebrations.

In Munich, West Germany, Drs Kugler and Laub have also looked at the effects of the weather on people with migraine. In six patients whom they studied for five years they found no correlation between the headaches and the atmospheric pressure, temperature, humidity or ionization (electrical charging of the air). But they did find a seasonal difference in the number of headaches. Fewer people had high scores in July, and the maximum number of headaches occurred in November and February. They also found an increase in complaints when major weather disturbances had just ended and a decrease when the weather was pleasant.

However, this could again be explained on a stress basis as there is no doubt that for most people bad weather creates more problems than good.

Hot dry winds

Professor F.G. Sulman in Jerusalem, Israel, thinks that hot dry winds are a cause of migraine and headache, and that the electrical charges (positive ionization) are responsible for this. The positive ionization caused by dust storms acts on a constituent of the blood to cause the release of a substance known as serotonin, which, as we have seen in chapter two, may bring on a headache.

The list of winds traditionally associated with headache reads like an exotic roll-call and includes the Foehn of the European Alps, the Mistral of France, the Sirocco of the Mediterranean, the Xlokk of Malta, the Chamsin or Sharav of the Middle East, the Santa Ana of California, the Chinook of Canada and the Zonda of Argentina.

In any atmosphere which is too dry there may be a preponderance of positively charged ions in the air and such conditions can occur in a stuffy, smoky room. Such an atmosphere may also bring on a headache or you may be like the university lecturer whose attacks were brought on by certain smells such as stale smoke, but particularly by perfume.

Smells

Fuad Assiz is a university lecturer from the Middle East. He came to me complaining of severe right-sided headaches which he had had for the last four years. The pain used to start on the right side of his nose, spread up to his right eye and then over the right side of his head. When asked what brought the headache on he said it was scent. On going into his history I discovered that if he met anyone who was wearing a heavy scent he developed a blocked feeling in the right side of his nose and this was followed by the headache.

He could not go into the perfume department of a large store because this invariably brought on his headache. He had found that on occasions he had been unable to continue his teaching if one of his women students was wearing scent and he said that this was particularly liable to happen in the morning when the scent was freshly put on.

Once, he had woken with a headache to find his wife dressed and ready to go out. He was sure that something must have brought on his headache and he asked her if she had been using scent; she admitted that she had. Usually she used toilet water only.

The only other thing that brought on his symptoms was stale cigar smoke. His case was unusual in that the trigger factor was a distinctive smell. His attacks were relieved by pain-killers and to a certain extent he could prevent them by taking a drug called metoclopramide if he knew that he was going into a heavily scented atmosphere.

Fuad Assiz was one of the lucky ones in the sense that there was something positive he could do to avoid an attack, but for many women all over the world migraine seems linked to factors over which they have no control.

Hormonal factors

Many more women than men have migraine and put briefly the reason appears to be the hormonal changes that occur in women. But the subject of women and migraine is of such importance that it needs a chapter on its own.

5 WOMEN AND MIGRAINE

As I have already pointed out, migraine and other headaches are three times more common among women than men. But both sexes have fewer headaches as they get older. The reasons for this are not fully understood. The fact that the difference in incidence of migraine between the sexes starts only after the age of eleven suggests a hormonal cause, but the difference continues up to the age of sixty or seventy by which time the hormonal changes which occur during the menstrual cycle are long since over.

Migraine and menstruation

It seems likely, however, that the action of the female hormones (oestrogen and progesterone) plays an important part in the migraine syndrome in some women. The menstrual cycle usually lasts for twenty-eight days and during the first two weeks the ovary prepares for the production of an egg cell. During this time the blood vessels of the uterus become larger, thicker-walled and more twisted and there are similar but less marked changes in some other blood vessels in the body.

If the egg, known as the ovum, is not fertilized the lining of the uterus is shed and menstruation takes place. For some women it is just before or at this time that headaches are most likely to occur.

The menstrual cycle is controlled by a delicate balance of hormones, the two main ones being oestrogen and progesterone. Oestrogen is secreted during the first half of the cycle and in the second half progesterone is secreted as well. If fertilization does not occur the progesterone secretion diminishes over a period of two weeks but if the woman becomes pregnant, progesterone continues to be secreted.

If you are asked whether your headaches occur when you have your periods you are very likely to reply yes. This is because you would probably include any headaches which came on during the week before your period or the week of the period, or just after it stopped – in other words, about 60 per cent of the twenty-eight-day menstrual cycle.

If the term menstrual migraine is limited, as it should be, to attacks linked to the first day of the period, it is found to be much less common, only occurring in about 10 per cent of migraine cases in women. With this kind of migraine it is often found that there is fluid retention at about the same time as the periods start.

A lot of medical research has been done into the hormonal patterns of migraine. Dr Somerville of Sydney, Australia, found that women with menstrual migraine have a similar hormonal pattern to other women but that the triggering factor in these people seemed to be a drop in the oestrogen level, not a change in the progesterone level as had been thought. He found that progesterone had no effect on the headaches but that they could be postponed if the oestrogen level was kept artificially high. Giving oestrogen to women during the first half of the cycle was, however, usually ineffective in preventing migraine.

Pregnancy

If you are expecting a baby you will probably find that your migraine is much better, with any luck you might be completely free of them for this period. The reason may be because instead of the regular rise and fall of the hormones during the menstrual cycle, there is a rise in the oestrogenic hormones, or it may be because of the biochemical changes that occur during pregnancy.

Betty Wells is aged thirty-five. She had her first attack of migraine when she was fourteen, about ten months after her periods started. The attacks were typical of classical migraine with a visual warning symptom of flashing stars, usually on the right side, followed by a left-sided headache, nausea and vomiting. She had about one attack a month and these responded well to pain-killers. About eighteen months ago she and her husband moved into a new house. While she was decorating and working hard to get the house in order her headaches became more frequent and began to occur about once a week. She came to see me at the Clinic on several occasions but there was very little change in her headaches.

About a year ago she came to me again saying that she was feeling very well and had not had a headache for two months. She also said that she was now three months pregnant. She remained headache-free until two months after the birth of her baby. From then on her headaches returned, although now she has only about one every two months and they are not nearly so severe.

The Pill

Headache is one of the commonest side-effects of the contraceptive pill and about 7 per cent of those taking it develop headaches. If you are taking one of the contraceptive pills this is one of the side-effects that your doctor will warn you about.

The headache is usually in the front part of the head and not very severe. It tends to come on the day after you stop taking the Pill and is called a release headache. This is not a type of migraine but is due to the Pill and most people find that it is relieved by simple pain-killers. It is most likely to occur if the Pill you are prescribed contains a high dose of oestrogen. Most of the modern contraceptive pills have only a low dose of oestrogen in them and some contain progesterone only.

If you suffer from migraine the Pill may occasionally make your headaches worse. If it does, you must tell your doctor, who will probably advise you to use some other form of birth control. On the other hand, there are a few people who find that their migraine is better when they are taking the Pill. If you do have migraine and you want to take the Pill you should consult your doctor for advice on the best one. Most likely you will experience no difficulties, but if your headaches do get worse on the Pill you should stop taking it.

Migraine and the menopause

Migraine tends to come on around the time of the first period and to get better after the menopause. There are several reasons for this. One is that, because the regular hormonal changes which occur during the menstrual cycle cease after the menopause, the levels of oestrogen and progesterone remain more or less constant. Another is that many people as they get older find life less stressful than they did in their twenties. A third possible reason is that in later life one's blood vessels become less sensitive to biochemical substances in the blood and are therefore less likely either to constrict or widen.

Oestrogen replacements which are sometimes prescribed during the menopause may bring on headaches. If this should happen tell your doctor and he will probably reduce the amount of oestrogens he is giving you and the headaches will improve. Although migraine symptoms often improve at the menopause, some people, I'm afraid, will continue to get headaches into their sixties and seventies. There is no evidence to suggest that removal of the womb, hysterectomy, helps migraine sufferers.

A number of women will probably find that the pattern of their migraine attacks changes over the years.

Like many migraine sufferers, Freda Travers has a history of being travel sick as a child. Her first memory of a migraine attack was when she was twelve, not long before her first period. These attacks persisted throughout her school life and tended to be worse when she was under stress, becoming much worse before her examinations.

After she left school her headaches improved for a few years but became worse in her late twenties. This was a time when there were considerable family difficulties: her father developed cancer and she helped her mother nurse him through his final illness. Her headaches at that time were occurring about every three weeks and she was losing at least one day a month from her work as a secretary.

When she first came to see me she said that she had 'tried everything' for her headaches but they did not seem to get any better. She also said that in addition to her migraine she now had other headaches which came on every day and which were like a band round her head. She was able to differentiate between the two quite different types of headache and was at that time suffering from a combination of migraine and tension headache.

I saw her at intervals during the next few years and during that time her tension headaches got much better but she still had migraine attacks. Her periods became irregular when she was forty-four and stopped when she was forty-five. After the menopause she had no further migraine attacks.

44

Not the vapours

During the nineteenth century migraine was regarded as an affliction of nervous women and was sometimes referred to as 'sick headache'. A bottle of smelling salts was often considered sufficient remedy and many women must have suffered unduly because no one took their headaches seriously. Even in this more enlightened century many men still prefer to refer to their headaches as hangovers rather than admit to having migraine.

One of the reasons why there has been so much difference of opinion about both the number of people with headache and the proportion of women sufferers to men was that until migraine was socially and medically accepted as a genuine disorder many men were unwilling to admit that they suffered from it. They were afraid they would be labelled malingerers or regarded as effeminate.

Indeed, it is only relatively recently that it has been widely recognized that migraine is an organic disorder which has a definite treatment.

The working woman

Many women today have full-time jobs and thousands more work part-time. This way of life has potentially made the woman's life more interesting and it certainly increases the family income. But trying to do two jobs is always a bit of a strain; and this is virtually what it amounts to as most working women also have a home and perhaps a family to look after. It is not surprising therefore that more women than ever now seem to suffer from headache.

Perhaps one of the reasons why I am interested in migraine and other kinds of headache is because I suffer from migraine myself. When I was a child the headaches were usually right-sided, and associated with vomiting. Very often they came on after going to the cinema particularly if I had to sit near the front (in those days the cinemas were aptly known as 'the flicks').

Recurrent headaches occurring once every one or two months became part of my life and I did not bother much about them. However, I well remember my first major visual symptom. It started with bright dancing lights on the right side of my field of vision and then slowly I lost the vision on that side. As I was a medical student at that time I immediately thought that I had a brain tumour and was very frightened. After about fifteen minutes normal v.sion returned and the headache and feeling of sickness started. The visual symptoms recurred on several occasions and over the years became less frightening.

Now that I am older I still get headaches, usually right-sided, the pain being in the right temple. They are always associated with nausea and sometimes with vomiting. The headaches tend to come on if I have been working too hard or if I have not had enough sleep for some reason such as travelling. Anti-sickness pills have been a great help to me because I know that if I take these and some simple pain-killer when the pain starts, the migraine proper will not develop. More recently I have developed attacks in which I get the visual symptoms only and which last from 15 to 45 minutes.

How your family can help

The mother is the linchpin of the family and if she is ill everything seems to go wrong; so if mother suffers from migraine, all the family are likely to be involved. Indeed, if any member of the family has migraine it is important that the rest of the family should know about it. Trying to hide a bad headache by carrying on as if nothing is wrong with you can be very difficult and in any case is not always the wisest course. On the other hand, no one should use their headache or any other disability to try to manipulate the rest of the family into doing what they want them to do.

So if you do have migraine how can your family help you? For a start they can make sure that you do not have all the work to do on your own. For instance, some help in getting ready for a vacation, such as taking the dog to the kennels or getting the clothes back from the cleaners, may make all the difference to being ready in time. All children make unreasonable demands on their parents at some time but if you can persuade your children to help, you are less likely to get over-tired.

When you do have a migraine try to get to bed for an hour or two when you have taken your pills because going to sleep will probably help you get better more quickly than anything else.

When you are lying down the family can help by bringing you a cup of tea and then getting on with their normal life without worrying you every five minutes for your advice, or demanding to know where the jam or the key of the tool shed is. Most migraine headaches, with the proper treatment, are better in a few hours so the family should try to give you relative peace for this length of time.

Your family should be discouraged from making too much noise, like playing records at high volume, but should not be kept unduly quiet because the most restful thing if you are unwell is to hear normal family life going on about you – total silence might make you anxious at the thought of what they might be up to!

In some families if the mother or father gets a headache, it is a time to be dreaded by everyone. But this should not happen. The one thing to remember when you have an attack of migraine is that however bad you feel at the time it will pass; and with the proper treatment you can learn to manage the headache. There is no need for everything to come to a standstill. Master your migraine – never let it master you. In the next chapter I will try to show you how.

6 WHAT CAN YOU DO TO HELP YOURSELF?

Keep a record

Although so far no cure has been found for migraine there are many ways in which you and your doctor can collaborate to reduce both the severity and the frequency of your attacks. You can also do some groundwork on your own.

The first thing is to try to find out if there is any particular situation or activity that brings on an attack. It can be very helpful to keep a diary in which you record the day and the time of the headache and also what you have been doing or eating for the previous twenty-four hours. You may find that you tend to get a headache if you have had an evening out. If you do, the headache may be brought on by the alcohol you have drunk; by being over-tired after going to bed much later than usual; by the excessive noise to which you may have been exposed – in a disco for instance; by the rich and unsuitable food you have eaten; or by the stuffy smoky atmosphere. Or, if you are a woman, perhaps your monthly period started on the morning of your attack.

For many people a combination of factors may start off a migraine attack and the actual cause or causes are not always easy to determine. I have discussed some of the commonest trigger factors in chapter four. Emotional or physical stress can bring on an attack. Although it is relatively easy to avoid physical stress – for example, by playing squash only if you are fit enough and by starting off gradually if you are taking up jogging or some other new activity – emotional stress is far harder to avoid. This is because it usually involves other people as well as yourself.

Don't go hungry

Migraines may be brought on by missing meals as well as by eating things which do not suit you. It is important that you should give yourself time to have a proper breakfast and not rush out to work after only a quick cup of coffee. If for any reason you should miss breakfast, try to have something to eat and drink during the morning.

Some schoolchildren tend to get up late and rush off without eating breakfast. It is important to see that this does not happen to your children, because not only might they get migraine but research has shown that children who go to school hungry do less well at their lessons. They also tend to have snack meals, perhaps spending their money on chocolate or potato chips, both foods which in themselves may bring on an attack.

Watch what you eat
The exact role of food in triggering off a migraine attack is still not clear. Sometimes it seems to be something in the food which usually or always brings on an attack, but it is also possible that migraine is part of an allergic reaction and this is more difficult to find out. The subject of food and migraine is discussed in detail on pages 30 to 35.

If you think that a certain food or drink may bring on an attack, keep a note of when you eat it and see if the headaches come on afterwards; then try to avoid that particular food or group of foods for some time – four weeks is generally considered to be about right. If your attacks stop completely or are much better, then you know that you have found the answer, but if there is no change in the pattern and severity of your headaches, that particular food can be reintroduced into your diet and you can try leaving out another one. However, if your headaches come on once every two or three weeks, you need to leave out that particular food for at least six to eight weeks before you can be sure whether or not it is making a difference.

Avoid extremes of temperature
Extremes of heat or cold can bring on a migraine attack, and although most of us do not get very cold, you may find that a cold swim or shower brings on a headache. If this applies to you, it is best to avoid very cold water. Over-exposure to the sun can also cause a headache and too much sun-bathing is unwise. Be particularly careful of the glare of the sun on sea or snow because bright, dazzling light can be another precipitating factor in a migraine attack. Some people may get relief by wearing dark glasses, but there is no advantage to be gained in wearing them all the time.

Hot dry weather, thunderstorms, snowstorms and sandstorms have all been linked by one sufferer or another to migraine but it is more likely that it is your reaction to these conditions and the stress they cause that brings on a headache, rather than the conditions themselves. There is no doubt that being caught in a storm can be very worrying and stressful.

Pain-killers

Aspirin and paracetamol (Acetaminophen in the United States) are two effective pain-killers which are available without a prescription in most countries and they have been used with great success over the years in the treatment of migraine. Aspirin is perhaps the best of the pain-killers; also, in feverish illnesses it brings down the temperature.

Although it is so readily available and cheap, don't forget that aspirin should be used with care and kept out of the hands of children. It must not be taken by anyone who has a history of indigestion as it can cause bleeding from the stomach and the gut. It should never be used by people taking anticoagulants (drugs which stop the blood clotting). The dose for adults is one to three pills (300 to 900 mg), taken up to a maximum of three times a day. Children should not be given aspirin because of the remote possibility of Reyes disease but should be given paracetamol instead. Calpol is a form which is suitable for small children.

Paracetamol (Acetaminophen) is usually the best treatment for those who cannot tolerate aspirin. Like aspirin, it was first used in the 1890s and over the last forty years has become a very popular analgesic. Although paracetamol has fewer toxic effects than aspirin it should be used carefully – as indeed should any drug which is pharmacologically active – because if too much is taken, as could be the case in a suicide attempt for instance, severe liver damage may occur and large amounts taken over long periods can damage the kidneys. The dose is two pills (1 g) with a maximum of 2 to 4 g a day for adults.

Sleep

Sleep is a necessary part of the recovery process in migraine and people who can lie down in a warm comfortable environment do better than those who stay up and try to work. Some people

OPPOSITE: The risk of migraine being started by bright sunlight – either direct, or reflected from surfaces like snow – can be lessened by wearing dark glasses.

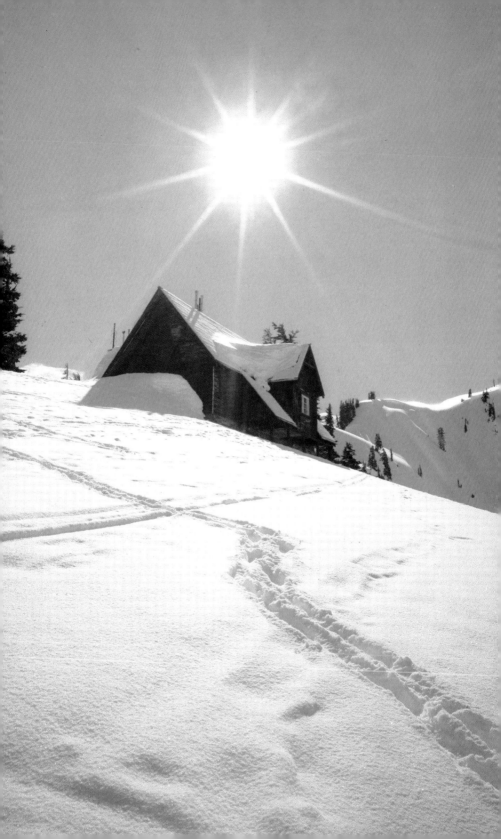

prefer to rest in an armchair or rocking-chair. Choose whatever is best for you, but remember that if you can go to sleep this will help you get over your headache more quickly.

At home

It is usually easier to cope with an attack when you are at home. The best thing to do is to take an aspirin or other pain-killer and go to bed for an hour or two. If you have small children to look after it may be safer and more convenient to lie down on the floor and let them play quietly around you; in fact they will probably take less notice of you if you do this than if you shut yourself away in the bedroom. Forget about the housework and the shopping until the attack is over.

Gentle massage
You may find that a throbbing head is eased by gentle massage, and if you are tense or under strain, soothing out the worry muscles on your forehead can be a help (see chapter twelve for illustrations of massage techniques). Quite a common finding in a migraine attack is pulsation of the temporal artery on one or both sides of the head. Pressing with the fingertips over the affected artery often relieves the pain, although it tends to recur when the pressure is released.

Hot and cold compresses
A cold compress can also be helpful, particularly if you feel flushed and your head is throbbing. A recent innovation are special pastes enclosed in plastic containers which can either be cooled in a refrigerator or warmed in hot water and then tied round the head. These have the advantage that they remain cool or hot longer than do the old-fashioned water compress and they do not drip. The contents are similar to those in the packs sold for keeping food cool. Most people find cold compresses are more soothing, but a few find hot ones better.

Learn to relax
It is a sad fact that stress and anxiety can bring on a headache but there are some simple exercises which you can do that will help you relax the muscles which get tensed up. You can easily do them at home.
     One way of finding out whether you are tense or not is to lie

on the bed and relax completely. Then ask a friend to try to remove the pillow. If when this is done your head is held rigid as if the pillow was still there, you are not relaxed and you may find the exercises described and illustrated in chapter twelve helpful.

A more sophisticated method of encouraging relaxation involves the use of electrical instruments which feed back a signal to the user. This is known as biofeedback, and is described in detail on page 101.

Meditation and yoga
Relaxation therapy can be combined with one of the techniques of transcendental meditation. These techniques were used successfully in Sydney by the Australian doctors, Dr G. Warner and Professor J.W. Lance. They found that if personal tuition was followed by the patient practising at home with the help of tape recordings of the instructor's voice, good results were obtained in people with chronic tension headache. It was less successful with people suffering from migraine.

There is no doubt that many people have found meditation and yoga helpful. To some extent you can always help yourself in or before an attack. By adjusting your way of life and by avoiding certain stressful situations you will probably be able to get some control over the frequency and severity of your attacks.

At work

If your headache comes on at work, it may not always be possible to lie down. However, if you have a sympathetic boss you may be able to sit somewhere quiet for a few minutes and take a pain-killer. In a mild attack you will probably be able to carry on with your work after a while, but if the attack becomes severe you will probably have to go and lie down. It is important that if you are taking any special pills that your doctor has prescribed for your migraine you should always have them with you in your pocket or handbag. 'Working through' an attack or taking stimulants such as caffeine is likely to prolong the headache, but some sufferers get relief from a cup of tea or other hot drink.

Noise, driving a car, riding a bicycle, or any other physical stimuli, may make your headache worse, so avoid them if

you possibly can. Driving at night when you have a migraine attack can be very dangerous, particularly if you experience any visual disturbances, as this could seriously impair your judgement. It is essential that you stop the car as soon as it is safe to do so and park by the side of the road, or preferably in a parking area. Get into the back seat, stretch out and try to rest or sleep until the attack wears off.

If you can learn to manage your migraine or your other headaches so that they do not interfere with your work or family life that is good, but if the situation gets out of hand remember that family doctors are there to help you. We will now look at their role in the treatment of your migraine.

OPPOSITE: Headlight glare and traffic jams on the way home from a hard day's work may precipitate a migraine. If your vision is ever disturbed during a migraine attack while driving, you must stop the vehicle and rest until your sight returns to normal.

7 HOW CAN YOUR DOCTOR HELP?

A very great number of headaches, including migraine, can be helped in the ways suggested in the previous chapter and it is certainly always worth trying them before going to see your doctor. If you find your headache is severe and persistent, or if you develop a different type of headache, you should go and see your family doctor. He will probably ask you all about your headache, how long you have had it, where the pain is, what brings it on, what makes it worse and if there is anything you know that helps it, and so on.

He may also ask you about your working conditions and family because as we have seen these can affect your headaches. After this he will probably examine you to make sure that apart from the headaches you are quite fit. Very often people are worried that headaches may be a symptom of a brain tumour and knowing that the doctor has examined them carefully and has found no sign of any disease relieves the tension and the headaches may improve.

Sometimes your doctor will suggest that you have special tests done. These usually include an X-ray of the skull and, nowadays, a brain scan. The type of scan done today is computerized axial tomography – the CAT scan. This is a complicated X-ray technique which will show if there is any abnormality in the brain. It is a quick and painless method of investigation but rather expensive so it is only carried out when there is some doubt about the diagnosis. People with migraine nearly always have normal results from CAT scans. Another investigation that your doctor may suggest is an electro-encephalogram. This is a technique by which the electrical activity of the brain can be recorded.

For most people with migraine, special tests are not necessary as the diagnosis can usually be made from the history and examination. Once the diagnosis has been made, your doctor will decide what treatment he thinks you need. Treatment can be given for the acute attack, or you may need both attack and preventive (prophylactic) treatment. If you have less than two attacks a month, treatment for the attack is probably all that you require.

Treatment of an acute attack

Relatively few patients are seen by their doctors while they are actually having a migraine attack. This may be because many attacks start early in the morning while the sufferer is at home in bed; or because migraine, although severe and disabling, is not a lethal disorder and therefore doctors are rarely called to a patient's home to give emergency treatment. Also, during an attack most people feel too ill to make the trip to the doctor's surgery.

When you get your migraine headache the one thing you probably want to do is lie down in a quiet room and if possible go to sleep. This should be the basis of any treatment of a migraine attack. But as the symptoms of an attack are nausea and vomiting, as well as headache, your doctor can help in prescribing an anti-sickness drug in addition to finding the best pain-killer for you.

Anti-sickness drugs

Doctors have found that the most effective anti-nauseant drug is metoclopramide (Maxolon or Primperan in Britain, Maxolon in Australia, Reglan in the United States, and Reglan or Maxeran in Canada) or a similar drug peridone (motilium). This drug not only stops the feeling of sickness but also tends to promote normal activity in the stomach, thereby increasing absorption of the pain-killer. Two preparations containing an analgesic together with metoclopramide have recently been introduced in Britain and Ireland (Paramax and Migravess). All these medicines can only be prescribed by a doctor.

Ideally, the anti-sickness pill should be taken as soon as the first symptom occurs, and the pain-killing drug ten to fifteen minutes later. The earlier in the attack you take the anti-sickness drug the more likely it is to be effective. The same applies to pain-killers.

Pain-killers

Aspirin and paracetamol (Acetaminophen in the United States), which have been used for many years in the treatment of migraine, are available without prescription. Nevertheless, as always, care should be taken in their use. As mentioned previously, aspirin should be avoided if there is a history of indigestion or gastric disturbance and should not be taken by those receiving anticoagulation treatment. Consult your doctor if you are in any doubt.

Some people are allergic to aspirin and may come up in a rash if they take it. They should ask their doctor for an alternative drug.

Sedatives

Anxiety or stress of any kind may bring on an attack of migraine and if you feel tense or anxious you may be helped by a sedative or muscle relaxant. One of the short-acting benzodiazepines, such as potassium clorazepate (clorazepate dipotassium in North America) may be prescribed. These are particularly helpful if you can lie down and go to sleep after taking one. Taking such a drug occasionally during an attack is not likely to cause habituation. A word of warning, however: they should never be taken if you have to drive, or operate heavy machinery as apart from making you feel drowsy they could impair your judgement.

It has been shown that people who sleep soundly during an attack do better than those who only rest or doze; because of this it is as well to avoid drinking strong coffee or taking any drug that contains a large amount of caffeine.

Ergotamine tartrate

Another drug that your doctor may prescribe is ergotamine tartrate. For the last thirty years this drug has been extensively used in the treatment of migraine. While it is undoubtedly helpful in a number of people, it is a very active drug pharmacologically and must be used with caution because unless care is taken symptoms of ergotamine tartrate poisoning may occur. These are nausea, vomiting, headache and a feeling of not being very well – in fact, symptoms very similar to those of a migraine attack. It is because of this similarity that over the years many people have inadvertently been taking too much ergotamine tartrate, thinking that because their symptoms have become worse, they require a larger dose.

There are many different preparations of the drug on the market available on prescription and this can lead to problems because it is quite possible to take several pills, each containing ergotamine tartrate, without realizing that they have the same contents. The following is a list of some common drugs containing ergotamine tartrate showing the quantity of active ingredients one pill from each preparation contains.

Cafergot (USA, UK, Canada, Australia)	ergotamine tartrate 1 mg caffeine 100 mg
Cafergot suppository (UK)	ergotamine tartrate 2 mg caffeine 100 mg
Ergomar (USA, Canada)	ergotamine tartrate 2 mg
Ergostat (USA)	ergotamine tartrate 2 mg
Lingraine (UK)	ergotamine tartrate 2 mg
Lingraine (Australia)	ergotamine tartrate 1 mg
Medihaler (UK)	ergotamine tartrate 0.36 mg per puff
Migral (USA)	ergotamine tartrate 1 mg cyclizine hydrochloride 25 mg caffeine hydrate 50 mg
Migral (Australia) and Migril (UK)	ergotamine tartrate 2 mg cyclizine hydrochloride 50 mg caffeine hydrate 100 mg

Ergotamine tartrate can also be taken by inhalation and the Medihaler ergotamine dispenses 0.36 mg of ergotamine tartrate per dose (0.45 mg in Australia).

Ergotamine tartrate is necessary for about one third of patients with migraine: between 1 and 2 mg per attack is all that is needed. In the past some people have taken 2 mg every night to try to ward off the headache which occurs in the morning, but this headache is not migraine but a result of an overdosage of ergotamine tartrate. The maximum amount of ergotamine tartrate taken in any one week should not exceed 6 mg. Therefore, those preparations which contain only 1 mg per tablet of ergotamine tartrate are preferable; if the effervescent tablets are used they should be cut in half, and only half a Cafergot suppository is necessary.

Daily headaches caused by ergotamine tartrate poisoning were at one time frequent but now this happens very much less often. It must be remembered that headaches which occur every day – apart from cluster headaches – are never due to migraine; the two commonest causes of daily headache being ergotamine tartrate poisoning and tension headache. The only time when ergotamine tartrate should be used every day is as a preventive drug in a bout of cluster headache.

Recently it has been shown that taking too many painkillers can cause headache. Anyone taking more than 16 painkillers per week for more than three months is likely to get analgesic abuse headache.

The pharmaceutical companies are now trying to find new drugs for the treatment of acute attacks of migraine. These are the 5HT agonists and antagonists. One of these, Sumatriptan, has now almost completed its clinical trials and it is hoped that this will be a useful addition to the treatment of an acute attack.

The sooner you get treatment the better

A study was done in 1976 on 310 patients who attended a London clinic for treatment of an acute attack of headache to try to find out what factors affected the rate and completeness of recovery. Each of the 310 patients attending the clinic was assessed and treatment was given according to their symptoms. Full records were kept of their attacks and of any headaches which occurred during the next seven days.

The possible factors which might affect the rate and type of recovery include the type of headache, the sex of the patient, the duration of the attack before coming for treatment, drugs taken prior to arrival at the clinic, the length and depth of sleep, and the length of stay. In this particular study no attempt was made to differentiate between the different types of treatment given in the clinic because what was considered to be the best treatment for each patient was given.

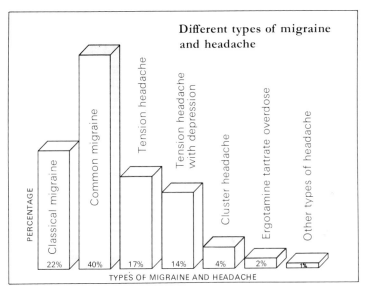

This graph clearly shows which type of migraine and headaches are most frequently experienced.

One aspect which could not be assessed was the therapeutic atmosphere, which in this study was the same for all patients. The following table shows the diagnosis in the patients.

The length of time the attack had been present before arrival at the clinic was noted in all cases and on the whole the patients who arrived early in an attack had significantly fewer headaches in the next few days than those who arrived after they had had the attack for twelve hours. 60 per cent of those coming when the headache had been present for less than six hours had no further headaches in the next seven days, while only 28 per cent of those who came when they had had a headache for more than twenty-four hours, were headache-free for the next seven days. The association between the time of arrival and recurrence of headache was more marked in those with tension headaches than those with migraine.

49 per cent of the patients slept either deeply all the time or intermittently while they were at the clinic, while the other half, 51 per cent, only rested or dozed. A significantly higher percentage of those who slept well recovered and were completely headache-free on leaving. This tendency was more marked in those with classical than with common migraine.

The average length of stay in the clinic was about three hours, ten patients staying for an hour or less. People were asked to say why they left and their replies were rather interesting. 2 per cent wanted to go before they were better because of business or social reasons. 17 per cent went before they were better because the clinic was closing. The majority, 79 per cent, chose to go because they were feeling better.

People were also asked what they had done on leaving the clinic. 26 per cent felt better and returned to work; 9 per cent returned to work with a slight residual headache; 45 per cent felt better but it was too late for them to return to work; and 19 per cent did not feel able to go back to work. In this survey no patients had attacks of migraine which went on for several days.

Preventive treatment

If you have more than two headaches per month preventive, or prophylactic, treatment may be necessary in addition to attack treatment. The first thing to do is to avoid, as far as possible, anything that is known to bring on an attack, as already mentioned in the last chapter. There are, of course, going to be some stresses which cannot be avoided but they can probably be minimized by careful planning. It is also important to avoid any food which is a known trigger factor. The drugs that your doctor might prescribe to prevent attacks can be divided into the following groups:

Anti-migraine drugs
There is a special group of drugs thought to have a particular action in migraine and known as 5HT antagonists. This group contains several of the commonly used preventive drugs, including pizotifen (pizotyline in Canada) and methysergide. Pizotifen (trade name Sanomigran in Britain, Sandomigran in Canada and Australia) works well for about a third of those who take it. The only unpleasant side-effects are drowsiness and weight gain. Methysergide (Deseril, or in North America the stronger Sansert) is closely allied to ergotamine tartrate and is effective in preventing attacks. But it does have several serious side-effects so is not recommended unless your migraine is very severe. Another similar drug is called dihydroergotamine.

A different sort of drug you may be prescribed in Great Britain or Australia is one called clonidine (Dixarit). This is useful in reducing the number and severity of attacks for about a third of people suffering from classical or common migraine. Its main side-effect is depression.

Beta-blockers have been used successfully in the treatment or prevention of migraine. Propranolol in doses of 40 mg two or three times a day is the one most often used to prevent attacks. This drug should not be taken if you suffer from severe chest or heart trouble. The unwanted side-effects can include depression, nausea and insomnia.

Dr Lee Kudrow has had considerable success in Encino, California, in treating cluster headaches with lithium, a drug sometimes used for depression.

Most of the drugs mentioned here can only be obtained on prescription, but even if you can get them over the counter you should not take them without consulting your doctor.

Anti-depressive drugs
People who have migraine are often depressed and although anti-depressants are not a treatment of migraine, your doctor may decide that you need a drug of this kind in addition to your migraine treatment. If you find that you are tired and anxious or have difficulty in sleeping – all possible signs of depression – go and see your doctor and he will advise you.

Acupuncture
This has become a very popular form of treatment in recent years. It can be given either by a doctor trained in acupuncture or by a non-medically qualified acupuncturist. The exact way in which acupuncture works is not known but there is no doubt that in some people the technique can relieve pain. However, it is unlikely that it can cure a specific disease. Its role in relieving migraine has not yet been fully assessed, but it seems likely that it is more useful in tension headache than in migraine.

Acupuncture
This has become a very popular form of treatment in recent years. It can be given either by a doctor trained in acupuncture or by a non-medically qualified acupuncturist. The exact way in which acupuncture works is not known but there is no doubt that in some people the technique can relieve pain. However, it is unlikely that it can cure a specific disease. Its role in relieving migraine has not yet been fully assessed, but it seems likely that it is more useful in tension headache than in migraine.

8 TENSION HEADACHE

Nearly all of us will have periods of anxiety and worry in our lives, whether it is caused by a love affair or a broken marriage, a sick child, business or financial troubles, or one of the thousand everyday problems which beset most of us at some time. So it is not surprising that tension or stress is one of the commonest causes of headache. Each year vast quantities of pain-killers are sold across the counter in supermarkets and pharmacies for the treatment of tension headache. And every year thousands of people go to their doctors seeking relief from the pain. Many more probably suffer in silence.

The pain

The pain of tension headache, unlike migraine, is usually dull and persistent, and can last all day, though its severity may vary. It is often described as a feeling of pressure or heaviness rather than pain and a common analogy is to a tight band round the head or a weight pressing down on top of the head. Sometimes the pain starts in the neck and then spreads up over the head.

When a headache is persistent it tends to get worse towards the end of the day, particularly if conditions at work have been difficult. Unpleasant physical conditions such as glare, poor lighting, or loud noise generally exacerbate it; they can also trigger it off.

Some people complain that their headache is there the whole time they are awake. Others wake up with a throbbing feeling in the head, but after getting up and having a cup of tea they find that the pain settles down to a dull ache.

Tension headaches are usually present all day and every day. In milder cases they develop during or after an obvious period of stress and then pass away once the strain of the situation has eased.

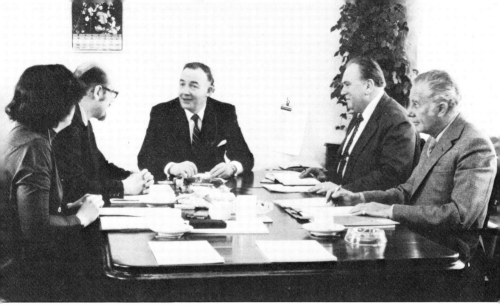

Tension headache brought on by the prospect of a tough business meeting is a common experience.

Drivers on their way to work may feel a headache coming on if they are held up in a traffic jam, and the slower and more trying the journey the worse the headache becomes. Some people get a headache if they have something unpleasant coming up such as a difficult meeting or an examination. Nineteenth-century author Lewis Carroll, who as we have seen suffered from headache himself, has Tweedledum say before his battle with Tweedledee in *Through the Looking-glass* (1872): 'I'm very brave generally, only today I happen to have a headache.'

If the headache is very severe, light may be unpleasant and many people who suffer from tension headache constantly wear dark glasses, even when they are indoors.

The following two examples are typical of a common pattern for tension headache.

Theo Wilde is the only son of elderly parents and has always been a very hard and conscientious worker. He was born in an industrial town and his father worked all his life in a textile mill. Theo won a scholarship to university where he obtained a creditable degree. Later he took a diploma in education and got a job as a schoolteacher. At the school where he taught he had difficulty in keeping his classes under control and was frequently going to the head-teacher for advice.

He had first suffered from headaches when he was at university.

When they started, the pain was dull and persistent, varying only a little in intensity during the day, then he began to experience sudden jabs of pain against a background of general discomfort. By the time he came to see me at the Clinic the pain was so bad that he was losing two days a month from school because of it.

His headaches were especially likely to come on at examination time when he was under pressure because of extra work. After careful examination, the only thing I could find wrong with Mr Wilde was tenderness in the muscles on the right side of the back of his neck.

Barbara Matthews is thirty-five and works as a secretary in a big publishing firm, where she has been for the last fifteen years.

Recently she had found her work increasingly difficult as she had got a new boss who did not like the way she did things. She has been liable to headaches all her life, but now she found that she was scarcely ever without one. The pain was like a band round her head and was made worse by noise or stress.

When she came to the Clinic she said that the headaches were becoming unbearable. She looked thin and tense and sat clasping and unclasping her fingers. I found nothing abnormal on examination and thought that she was probably suffering from tension headache. Barbara had been worrying as to whether the headaches were due to a brain tumour and when I reassured her about this, for the first time during the interview she smiled. I prescribed some pain-killing drugs and showed her how to do some relaxation exercises. When she came back to the clinic a month later she was looking much better and although she was still having some headaches they were not causing her nearly so much discomfort.

Signs of tension

Some patients who come to our Clinic complaining of tension headache show signs of muscle over-contraction. Their forehead is wrinkled and there is contraction of the muscles of the jaw and temples. Sometimes the patient looks taut and anxious and he may clench and unclench his hands or move his fingers

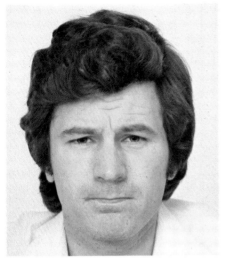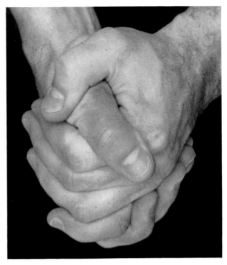

A wrinkled forehead, and wringing your hands are both signs of tension.

restlessly. Many people are tense without realizing it, and they may wonder why they feel so tired at the end of a day and why their muscles ache. In such cases, it is often very helpful to learn to relax.

Relaxing can be difficult

It is not always easy to relax and various exercises have been designed to help you in the task. The more anxious you are the harder it is and simple measures such as massage, gentle stretching of the neck and shoulders, and hot baths should all be tried. These and other ideas for relaxing are illustrated in chapter twelve.

Meditation, yoga and hypnosis have also been found helpful by some, as well as biofeedback conditioning techniques (see page 101). The biofeedback methods have generally employed feedback messages from the muscles of the forehead or temple. If you find this form of treatment beneficial you can continue it at home.

As well as lessening or abolishing the pain of the headache, relaxation of the muscles of the body can be very soothing both mentally and physically.

Psychological factors

These probably play a part in tension headache and many psychologists have found that there is a history of anxiety-provoking situations in a number of their patients. Conversely, the constant nagging pain of a tension headache may make you depressed. If you do feel depressed you should go and see your family doctor and he may decide that you need some treatment for it.

Listen to your doctor

Your doctor's attitude towards you is a very important part of the treatment he gives you and if you do not believe what he says he is unlikely to be able to help you. The first thing you want to know is what is wrong with you – have you got a serious illness such as a brain tumour? After he has examined you he will be able to reassure you on this point and you can then talk to him about your problems. He will probably explain to you the mechanism of your headache including the trigger factors. He is unlikely to be able to give you a permanent cure, but he may well be able to diminish the number and severity of the headaches.

Find the right pain-killer
When the pain is severe most people need some kind of pain-killer and, as in the case of migraine, aspirin or paracetamol (Acetaminophen) are the drugs most widely used. But some people prefer codeine or some other analgesic, or a proprietary combination of two or more analgesics. Once you have found a pain-killer which suits you it is best to keep to it, but it is important not to take too many.

Possible causes
It has been suggested that some of the pain in tension headache is caused by the narrowing or constricting of the small blood vessels supplying the muscles of the head and neck. There is no underlying structural damage to the brain nor are there, as far as we know, any underlying biochemical changes.

Sometimes the pain of tension headache is helped by substances such as alcohol or nicotinic acid because these widen the blood vessels. However, this does not mean that a large gin and tonic or a beer is the answer. At best a drink may bring temporary relief, but at worst it could bring on a more severe headache, and several drinks could result in the hangover headache, as you will see in the next chapter.

9 OTHER HEADACHES

The previous chapters have dealt with migraine and tension headache, but there are many other kinds of headache. We shall look here at some of the most common ones.

Hangover headaches
After drinking alcohol, especially if you have too much, you may wake up the following morning with a severe headache which is worse when you move and is often accompanied by feelings of malaise, nausea and fatigue. These unpleasant sensations usually last about five hours and then gradually wear off. Many drinkers think that some drinks such as brandy or red wine are more likely to cause a hangover than others, such as vodka; but it seems probable that it is the amount of alcohol consumed that is important. Many sufferers from migraine drink very little, if any, alcohol as they find that it can bring on an attack; this is particularly noticeable in those who suffer from cluster headaches.

'Chinese restaurant' syndrome
This type of headache is caused by a food additive, monosodium glutamate. The pain is usually in the forehead or temple and there may be a feeling of tightness round the face. Some people also complain of dizziness, feeling sick, diarrhoea or abdominal pain. Monosodium glutamate is one of the ingredients of soya sauce and is used as a food additive because of its flavour-enhancing properties.

The symptoms often come on after eating a Chinese meal and therefore have been called the 'Chinese restaurant' syndrome. Small amounts of monosodium glutamate will bring on a headache in susceptible people, particularly if taken on an empty stomach, and food containing this substance should be avoided. A 200 ml portion of *wun tun* soup is said to contain about 3 g of monosodium glutamate.

American researchers have shown that injections of monosodium glutamate in healthy volunteers can cause a burning or scorching feeling in the chest which spreads to the neck, shoulders, arms and abdomen. This is followed by a sensation of pressure and tightness in the chest which later spreads over the cheeks and radiates to behind the eyes. Other research has shown that symptoms appear after taking between 1.5 and 12 g of monosodium glutamate and that thresholds of 3 g or less are found in people who have these symptoms after eating Chinese food.

'Hot-dog' headaches

If you like frankfurters, bacon, ham or salami you may have experienced what has become known as the 'hot-dog' headache. It occurs as a result of eating cured meats such as those mentioned above. The headache usually occurs at the front of the head and is throbbing in character. It comes on about half an hour after eating the food. Often there is flushing and redness of the face and this is caused by chemicals called nitrites which are used in the curing. Some time ago it was found that the addition of sodium nitrite gave a uniform red colour to the meat. However, nitrites are known to widen the blood vessels and it is this which leads to the throbbing headache.

This type of headache is not migraine, but people with migraine are perhaps more likely to be vulnerable to the effects of nitrites in these foods than those who never have headaches.

'Ice-cream' headache

This is the type of sharp pain which occurs after eating ice-cream or other cold substances. It is probably due to excessive stimulation of one of the nerves in the head. Keeping ice or ice-cream in the mouth may cause immediate local pain in the palate or throat and later pain in the side of the face or the head. The cause of the pain is probably the sudden cooling of the mouth or throat because ice-cold objects in the gullet or the stomach do not cause this type of pain.

Dr Neil Raskin's research in San Francisco, California, shows that people prone to migraine are three times more likely to suffer from 'ice-cream' headache than those who are not prone to migraine, and that the former group's headaches are more severe.

However tempting they might look, ice-creams are best avoided by migraine sufferers as they are far more likely than most to develop the sharp pain of 'ice-cream' headache.

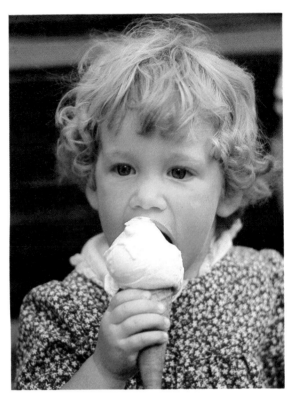

Explorers' headache

For over a hundred years Arctic explorers have written of the severe headache which they experience from time to time. Some of these headaches are undoubtedly migrainous but a few are due to eating too much vitamin A. Explorers in the Arctic were often invited to a meal by the Eskimos, and one of the delicacies which was usually served was polar bear liver. This contains an enormous amount of vitamin A (about 15,000 international units per pound; seal and halibut liver contain similar quantities).

Headaches caused by an excessive intake of vitamin A are usually focussed in the front of the head and behind the eyes, and are often associated with sickness, stomach-ache, vertigo, and lassitude. Usually these symptoms do not come on for at least four hours after eating.

In a study of four adult volunteers American scientists have found that 2 million units of vitamin A in a single dose caused dull headaches. Another American study described six patients who had daily pulsating headaches in the front of the head which came on days and even weeks after starting a regime that included taking 25,000 international units of vitamin A daily. These headaches cleared up after a few weeks when the excessive intake was stopped. Most people do not take these enormous amounts but children are particularly sensitive to overdoses. Substantial quantities of vitamin A occur in kidney, liver, fish liver oils and raw carrots, among other foods.

Mountain sickness (altitude headaches)
Mountain sickness has been known for over four hundred years. The symptoms, which include headache, nausea, dimness of vision, breathlessness, palpitations, loss of appetite and sleeplessness, usually occur only above 8,000 ft (2,400 m), and with increasing frequency at higher levels. The headache, which is throbbing and generalized, is made worse by jolting or coughing and relieved by lying down. It is likely that the headache and feeling of nausea are caused by lack of oxygen because in the early stages breathing pure oxygen brings relief. The symptoms usually take between six hours and three days to develop and improve when the sufferer returns to a normal altitude.

Headaches and sex
Happily, for most people sexual intercourse is not a cause of headache but there are two kinds of headaches which may be associated with sexual activity. In the first and commonest type the pain is in the back of the head and comes on as sexual excitement increases. The type of pain is probably due to excessive contraction of the muscles of the neck and head, and can be relieved or prevented by deliberately relaxing these muscles. The second type of headache is more severe, coming on immediately before or at the moment of orgasm, and is probably related to the rise in blood pressure which happens at this time. Anyone who gets a severe headache during or just after intercourse should consult his or her family doctor.

Headaches and serious illness

A sudden severe headache, particularly if followed by weakness of a limb, some disturbance of sensation or impairment or loss of consciousness, raises the fear that it may be caused by a serious disorder. Conditions which can start with a headache include meningitis, brain haemorrhage, brain tumour, sinusitis, feverish illnesses and temporal arteritis.

The headache in meningitis or encephalitis comes on rapidly, often in a few hours, and extends over the whole head and down the back. There is usually a high fever as well. Any movement tends to make the headache worse. If you get any of these symptoms you should immediately consult your doctor.

Brain tumour

People with severe and recurrent headaches are often afraid to go and see their family doctor because they think that they may have a brain tumour, but this occurs in only a tiny minority of cases.

Professor J.W. Lance and his colleagues studied a series of 1,152 patients who attended their headache clinic in Sydney, Australia, and they found that less than 1 per cent had a brain tumour.

The history of someone with a brain tumour differs considerably from that of someone with migraine. The sufferer is usually over the age of fifty, the headaches occur over a short period – probably less than three months – the pain is generally in the same place and is aggravated by bending, coughing, sneezing or other exertion. The headaches tend to be worse in the morning and get progressively more severe without the symptom-free periods which occur in migraine. There may be sensory disturbance or weakness in a limb, and drowsiness or fits may develop. If any of these symptoms occur you should go and see your family doctor as soon as possible. He will examine you and if necessary arrange special investigations which may include a CAT scan (see page 56). This type of X-ray will show whether you have a tumour or not.

Strokes

According to American physicians, just under a third of people who have a stroke have a headache just before the onset. The headache usually passes off after a few hours although other symptoms, which also come on beforehand, such as weakness or unsteadiness of a limb and sensory or visual disturbances, may persist.

Temporal arteritis

This is a rare disease of the arteries in the temples of the head which occurs in some elderly people. Often the first sign of the condition is pain over the arteries in the temple; these later become thickened and it is difficult to feel the pulse there. The skin over the affected artery may become red and very tender to touch. Headache is a common symptom and may be on one side of the head or on both sides, depending on which artery is involved, and chewing can be painful.

It is important to go and see your doctor if you have this type of disorder because it can normally be treated with drugs called steroids. If you do not get the proper treatment your vision may be affected.

Trigeminal neuralgia

This causes a very severe pain which occurs in bouts, and is sometimes confused with cluster headache (see page 8). The pain is felt over most of the face.

Each attack of pain can last for two to three hours in bouts of twenty to thirty seconds and continue over weeks or even months. Characteristically the person avoids stimulating the affected region in any way and sometimes omits to wash or shave that part of his face. It is not unusual to see an otherwise well-turned-out individual with one side of the face encrusted with dirt and the other side clean. Like cluster headache, trigeminal neuralgia tends to affect those over forty.

Sinusitis

Sinusitis used to be a diagnosis often made when people complained of headache, but the actual infection of a sinus happens comparatively rarely. If a sinus is infected there is pain and tenderness in that area. If the affected sinus is the frontal, or maxillary, one, bending forward or blowing your nose will make the pain worse.

Sinus pain is usually relieved if the obstruction blocking the sinuses is drained. Nose drops or a nasal spray may help to clear your nose and when the airway is clear you may find steam inhalation helpful. If the infection does not clear up after these simple measures it may be necessary to see your family doctor who may decide to give you antibiotics.

Chronic sinusitis is often blamed for vague discomfort in the forehead, across the nose or between the eyes, but most often the cause is muscle contraction; in other words, tension headache.

Blood pressure and headaches

Most doctors agree that a sudden rise in blood pressure can cause headaches. These headaches are usually on both sides, either at the front or the back of the head, and are commonly severe and bursting or throbbing. But it is doubtful whether a moderate rise in blood pressure, known as hypertension, causes headache. The normal blood pressure does not exceed 145/90 millimetres of mercury (the first number being the pressure recorded when the heart contracts; the second, when it relaxes), and any reading over this denotes a mild hypertension. It has recently been put forward that it could be the worry and stress over knowing you have high blood pressure rather than the blood pressure itself which causes the headache.

Dr Harold G. Wolff, an American doctor from New York, showed that the headaches of hypertensive patients responded well to rest and relaxation although there was no significant change in their blood pressure. People who have been told that they have raised blood pressure often become anxious and as a result may develop a tension headache.

A group of Scottish doctors studied a hundred patients and came to the conclusion that headache did not occur in those with mild or moderate hypertension, but that it was significantly more common in those with severe hypertension. When these patients' blood pressure dropped after treatment, their headaches improved.

Head injury

Head injuries of one kind or another happen fairly frequently. They range in severity from the mild bump suffered after walking into the kitchen cupboard to the severe trauma that may result from a traffic accident. Although it is a commonly held belief that a blow to the head causes a headache, this is probably true only in the short term. A headache from a minor knock usually goes after an hour or so, especially if you rest and take a pain-killer. Whether or not more severe head injuries cause periodic headaches over a number of months or years is open to question. Many people who have had relatively minor head injuries – namely those who have either not been unconscious or been unconscious for only a few seconds, or a minute or two at most – have taken legal action claiming that following their injuries they have been unable to work because of difficulty in concentration, headache, nausea, dizziness and other symptoms. Pain is a subjective thing and there is no doubt that some of these claims are true. But whether the pain or other symptoms are due to the actual injury or to the anxiety or worry which follow an accident, it is more difficult to say. There have been many cases in which the headache following an injury has improved dramatically after the legal case has been settled.

People who have suffered very serious head injuries, that is to say those who have been unconscious for a week or more, generally do not suffer from severe headaches. In fact, the number of headaches among people with serious head injuries is slightly lower proportionately than the number in the population as a whole – a very different picture from those with relatively minor head injuries.

The interesting question is why those who have severe head injuries do not suffer from headache. Possibly their other injuries, such as a broken leg, are so painful that they do not notice the headache. It could be that unlike those recuperating at home, whose anxieties about possible brain damage go unanswered, they are relaxed by the reassurance and care of expert hospital staff. Or it could be that the headache occurs during the time they are unconscious.

One particular group of very severely injured patients was monitored for two years and fewer than 10 per cent developed headaches of any kind. Again, this is less than the number of headaches in the general population. Occasionally, migraine can come on for the first time after a head injury but this is very unusual and headaches are more often of the tension type.

If you have had a head injury and get headache immediately after it, you should rest in bed until the headache is gone, because getting up and trying to do things too soon after an injury is very unwise. Anyone who has been involved in a car accident will know that driving a car again after the accident is difficult, partly because of the fear that another accident may occur, and partly in some cases because of the feeling of guilt, particularly if someone else has been injured. It is better to wait until you are feeling completely recovered before driving again. Anyone who falls off a horse is usually told to mount again immediately and ride on but this is probably also unwise.

Neck injuries

The whiplash car injury is nowadays a fairly common accident. It tends to occur when one car crashes into the back of another. In the front car the driver's head is forced forward and then jerks back over the car seat. It is very common in this sort of accident to sustain some damage to the muscles of the neck and, if it is severe, to the cervical spine itself. The pain is usually felt in the neck but later it may spread up over the back of the head. This type of pain is usually a constant nagging ache, made worse by movements of the head and neck, and in the first instance is usually due to spasm of the neck muscles. If the damage is to the cervical spine there may be rupture of one of the cervical discs.

Contrary to popular belief it is extremely difficult for the spine to be dislocated or get out of alignment because the cervical vertebrae are constructed in such a way that they overlap sideways and from front to back, and are held very firmly together by a complicated network of ligaments. If neck pain does come on after injury the best treatment is lying flat in bed and taking pain-killers.

It is only if the pain spreads down the arm or if there is weakness of the arms or legs that you should suspect a more serious injury; but wherever the pain, if it persists the family doctor should be consulted.

When the pain has subsided it is important that active exercises for the neck muscles should be done as most of the pain is caused by muscle spasm, which, after an initial period of rest, is most likely to be improved by active movements of the neck. If there is a fracture or fracture dislocation of one or more of the bones of the neck it may be necessary to wear a cervical collar for a short while under the direction of the doctor. It is, however, a bad idea to wear a cervical collar for a long period because having the neck held still may lead to a wasting away of the neck muscles. In fact, many of the collars that people wear are of very little value anyway as they are made of soft materials such as felt which do not immobilize the neck; if a collar does not keep the neck still there is very little point in wearing it.

10 CHILDREN AND HEADACHES

Headache is a very common part of many childhood illnesses and anyone who has had a child with mumps or measles knows that one of the earliest signs may be headache. The child often rubs his head saying that it feels funny and that it aches. The pain is usually felt in the front of the head. With the headache the child is often fractious and difficult to amuse, and generally does not want to eat anything. There is usually a fever and the temperature can go up as high as 102 or 103°F (39–40°C).

These are the sort of symptoms that we are all accustomed to when our children have one of the common infectious diseases. Once the spots of measles or whatever it is develop, the diagnosis is relatively easy; but it is in the early stage that headache in a child may be worrying.

When your child has an illness of this sort it is as well to call the doctor, but while he is on the way put your child to bed,

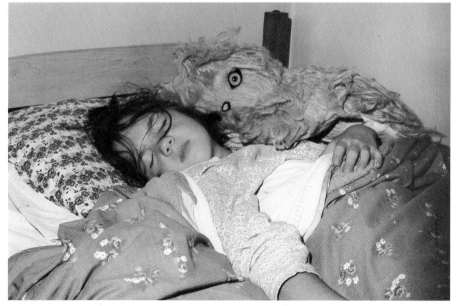

Children feverish with mumps or measles often complain of headache.

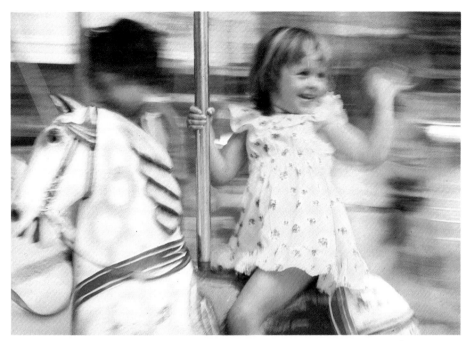

Children get migraine too. As with adults it can be triggered off by over-excitement.

keep him warm, do not bother trying to make him eat but encourage drinking as much as possible. It is particularly important for a feverish child to have a lot to drink. At this stage your child should be given a small dose of paracetamol and this will probably be enough to relieve the pain and help bring down the temperature. When the doctor comes, if it is an infection, he may prescribe the appropriate antibiotic with aspirin or paracetamol (Acetaminophen) as a pain-killer. Generally this kind of headache will go once the right treatment is given.

Migraine among children

If headaches do recur from time to time, especially if they are brought on by excitement – such as going to a party, or the theatre or going on vacation – and are associated with a feeling of sickness, they are probably due to migraine. These headaches are usually at the front of the head, sometimes on one side sometimes the other, and often the child will say that he doesn't feel well and doesn't want to eat. He may complain of feeling sick and occasionally he may vomit. If these attacks occur repeatedly and there are no other symptoms, a diagnosis of migraine is almost certain. But if you can conceal your anxiety your child will not be alarmed and very often the symptoms can be dealt with by a simple pain-killer such as paracetamol (Acetaminophen). For children over a year old 2.5-5 ml of Calpol is probably all that is required.

If nausea or sickness plays a big part in the symptoms it is sometimes necessary to give an anti-sickness medicine and for this small doses of a drug such as metoclopramide (see page 57 for trade names) may be prescribed. Metoclopramide may, however, cause extra pepamidal symptoms (jerking movements) if given to children under the age of fourteen. Parents should always be warned of this possibility and told not to give a further dose if this should happen.

The visual symptoms which occur in classical migraine are relatively rare in children. However, if they do come on they can be very frightening to a child, and if your child complains that he sees funny things, try to reassure him. Get him to tell you what they are like and where they are. He may say that he sees flashes of light or that there is a wavy light in front of his eyes, or even that he cannot see things properly. Sometimes he will tell you that this happens only on one side and that he can see clearly on the other. It is most helpful to your doctor if you can get a description of these symptoms because it will assist him in making a diagnosis of migraine.

Tummy aches

Sometimes a child will complain of feeling sick and of pain in the tummy at the same time as the headache; and in fact this pain may be the main complaint. If so, it is easy to mistake the illness for an abdominal disturbance such as appendicitis, or some other gastro-intestinal problem; and unfortunately in the past many children have had an operation for a grumbling appendix when in fact the pain was due to migraine. To avoid this happening it is very important to tell the doctor all the symptoms, particularly in the case of very young children who may find it difficult to talk to the doctor themselves. You should tell the doctor just how often your child has had similar attacks, if anything has brought on the attacks, such as excitement or emotional stress, how long they have lasted and if there are any other symptoms present.

Once a diagnosis of migraine has been established the doctor will explain that although migraine is an unpleasant condition it can easily be treated and that there is no serious underlying illness. However, a number of children who suffer from these abdominal symptoms do develop either common or classical migraine when they grow up.

What type of child has migraine?

It has been said that migraine affects the intelligent obsessive type of child but, as we have already seen in adults, there is very little evidence to support this theory. A Swedish study compared the personality and characteristics of a group of children with migraine with those of their fellows and no demonstrable difference in social class, intelligence, or ambition was found between the two groups. The study also showed that in children more boys than girls suffer from migraine although in adults, classical and common migraine are much commoner in women than in men.

Another finding suggested that there was no difference in the frequency of such symptoms as nail-biting, bed-wetting or nervous tics in children with migraine and children without, but that there was a slightly higher occurrence of sleep disturbance, temper tantrums and night terrors in the migrainous children. On the whole, the children with migraine seemed to be more tense, sensitive and vulnerable to any kind of frustration than other children.

Harry is the only child of Tom and Margaret. Tom is a keen sportsman who has never had a headache in his life, but Margaret has suffered from migraine since the age of twelve. Harry was a healthy baby but one day when he was about three, he became very angry when his mother insisted on bathing him when he wanted to go on playing with his toy bricks. He screamed and cried and when Margaret took his temperature she found it had risen alarmingly. She immediately called the family doctor who, apart from the raised temperature, could find nothing wrong with Harry. He prescribed some Calpol and the boy went to sleep and woke up his usual self in the morning. Over the next few months Margaret noticed that when Harry was upset or thwarted his temperature often did go up and he said his head hurt. These attacks were migrainous in nature and responded to treatment with simple pain-killers.

When Harry was a little older he started to be car-sick. This proved to be quite a problem until Margaret took him to the family doctor again and this time he was given anti-sickness pills in addition to the pain-killers, and Margaret was advised to give him these a few hours before the start of a journey. Margaret found that it was a good idea to have plenty of cool drinks with her as well as a supply of water, and a bucket and sponge should Harry be sick. She also encouraged him to run about and play whenever there was a break in the journey.

Travel-sick children sometimes develop migraine when they grow up, but with the right treatment Harry should be able to minimize the severity of his attacks and lead a normal life.

Tension headaches among children

Children as well as adults can get tension or muscle contraction headache. They usually come on when the child is under physical or emotional strain. For example, they might occur if there is an unhappy situation at home, such as strife between the parents. The child may also find that if he complains of headache and gets his mother's attention he can use them to manipulate the situation.

If a child is kept at home when he has a headache he may use his symptoms regularly to help avoid going to school, especially if he is unhappy there.

Have a word with the teacher if you think your child is having problems at school and make sure that there is someone at the school to give him any medication if he gets a headache during school hours.

If your child's headaches do not improve you should consult your doctor.

Children and their environment
Children may be able to manipulate the immediate situation but they cannot alter their environment and studies have shown that environmental factors in a particular area or region may influence the number of headaches.

An interesting study of headaches and migraine among schoolchildren in the northern Finnish community of Enontekiö was carried out by Drs Sillanpää and Peltonen. This was one of a

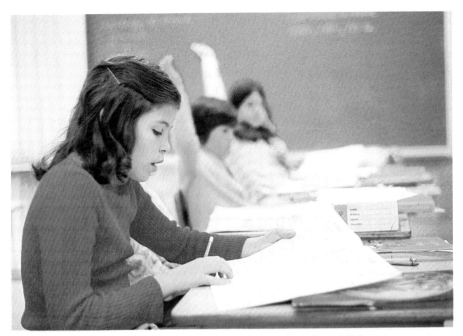

Problems at school can lead to tension headaches for children.

few scattered communities in Finnish Lapland where the range of weather and temperature during the year is extraordinary. During the summer the sun does not set for seventy days and there is no sunrise for fifty-six days in winter. The temperature varies between −58 and +86° F (−50 and +30° C).

In this study a questionnaire was sent to the families of pupils aged seven to fifteen years attending school in Enontekiö to find out how many children suffered from headache and migraine. It is interesting to compare Dr Sillanpää's and Dr Peltonen's figures with those of a similar survey conducted earlier in Sweden by Dr Bo Bille. The results of both surveys show a high number of headaches among the children – much higher than the average for children in the rest of the Western world.

		Sweden 1962	Lapland 1977
Aged 0–7 years	Headaches	57%	47%
	Migraine	1%	1%
Aged 7–15 years	Headaches	59%	61%
	Migraine	4%	4%

Fortunately, most of the headaches which occur in children do not have a serious underlying cause and can generally be treated by simple pain-killers. But, very occasionally, they may be an early symptom of a more serious disorder.

Serious illness

If your child gets an unexplained headache and then develops other symptoms such as stiffness of the neck, a drooping eyelid, or an epileptic fit you should immediately seek medical advice. Meningitis, encephalitis (inflammation of the brain) and brain tumour are all serious illnesses which can start with a headache. If you have any doubt about your child's symptoms always consult your doctor.

Keep all medicines out of reach

If the doctor prescribes any medicines or pills for you or your child do make sure that they are kept in a safe place, preferably a locked cupboard. Children, especially enquiring toddlers, tend to put everything into their mouths and this of course could, and sadly sometimes does, have dangerous consequences. Most young children are amazingly inventive in finding ways to get to high shelves so any medicines you have in the house should be put safely out of reach. Some pills come in 'child-proof' containers which is a sensible practice. Be especially careful with medicines which are sweet tasting or fruit flavoured. Many pills even look like candy sweets which of course makes them particularly tempting for small children.

11 RESEARCH AND MIGRAINE CLINICS

Migraine is not a killing disease and does not have the emotional appeal of heart transplant surgery, for instance. It is therefore less well funded. However, a considerable amount of research into migraine is going on and taking a number of interesting directions.

Distribution

One of the first things to establish about any disorder is who does it affect, how many people have it, how frequent are the attacks, and what, if any, are the precipitating or trigger factors. This is known by doctors as the epidemiology of the condition.

Professor W.E. Waters from the University of Southampton, England, has done a great deal of research into the epidemiology of headache and migraine in Britain, and it is interesting to look at some of his findings. Some of his earlier studies were done in Wales using a questionnaire which asked for details about headaches. The word migraine did not appear on the questionnaire, but everyone who had had a headache in the year preceding the survey was asked about migrainous features.

Professor Waters found that some features of migraine were surprisingly common among those with headache. He estimated that in an industrial valley in south Wales 19 per cent of all women aged between twenty and sixty-four had had migraine at some time in the year before the survey. He went on to say, however, that migraine is a difficult condition to define.

Professor Waters and his colleagues have since done studies on headache and migraine in a London general practice, in the Scilly Isles off the coast of Cornwall, in a prison, in two schools, and in an English city – Southampton. His conclusions are that headaches are commoner among women than men and that for both sexes the number declines with age. In Southampton he found that 73.1 per cent of the men and 81.4 per cent of the women had had a headache in the previous year, but only 12 per cent of the men and 19 per cent of the women had consulted their doctor because of it.

This work is important because not only does it show how widespread headache is, but it also emphasizes the fact that only a small proportion of people seek medical advice.

Research on blood flow

Whatever the underlying cause of a migraine attack may be, there is no doubt that the blood vessels are affected at some stage in the process. A great deal of research has therefore consisted of studies of the blood flow and the reaction of the blood vessels during and between attacks. Although there may be some difference in the blood vessels of people with migraine in the periods between the attacks, the main changes are always going to be during the attacks and it is for this reason that most research must be done at this time.

For many years it was thought that in the initial or early warning stage of the migraine attack the blood vessels constricted, that is to say they became narrowed, giving rise to the symptoms of the aura, and that the subsequent headache was due to dilation of these vessels. Recent work by Professor J Olesen of Copenhagen and his colleagues using xenon 133 by intra-arterial injection to measure regional cerebral blood flow, showed that there was a regional hypoperfusion i.e. a diminished blood flow. This developed before, and persisted throughout, the headache phase. This hypoperfusion probably reflected a disturbance of brain metabolism which was the cause of the symptoms and the pain of the headache was due to the production of substance P. This is an important group of studies as they suggest that the initial stages in a migraine attack are neuronal (in the brain cells rather than the blood vessels), and that the changes in the blood vessels are secondary.

In recent years new techniques such as infra-red cutaneous thermography and Doppler ultrasonography have been used to explore the activity of the smaller blood vessels of the head during an attack of migraine or cluster headache. Thermography is a technique by which changes in the skin temperature can be recorded. When the blood flow to an area increases, the temperature of the skin rises. The Doppler technique involves putting an ultrasonic transceiver over a blood vessel and by this method measuring the direction, velocity and turbulence of the blood flow in that vessel.

Other methods of investigating the changes in the blood circulation in the head are by studies of the blood flow in the brain and by cerebral angiography. In cerebral angiography radio-opaque dye is injected into one of the blood vessels and X-rays taken. Such X-ray pictures – called angiograms – have from time to time been obtained by chance during migraine auras, headaches or cluster headaches and none of these has shown any gross abnormality in the main blood vessels. This suggests that any change in size that occurs does so in vessels which are too small to be seen by this technique.

Biochemical research

The body is a very complex organism and all actions and reactions are associated with biochemical changes. Humans are the only animals known to suffer from headaches, so all direct observations on headache have to be done in humans; although some studies such as the reaction of arteries to certain substances can be done in other animals.

As we have seen, stress in any form may bring on a migraine attack and under stressful conditions the body produces substances known as catecholamines. These are hormones released by the adrenal glands and include adrenalin, noradrenalin and dopamine. Adrenalin and noradrenalin cause the heart to beat faster and prepare the body in times of danger. All three substances have a marked effect on the blood vessels and research is being carried out into the levels of these substances found in people during a migraine attack.

In the early 1960s Professor Federigo Sicuteri of Florence, Italy, found that during an attack, migraine sufferers had an abnormally high level of a substance called 5-hydroxyindole-acetic acid (5HIAA) in their urine. This is a breakdown product of serotonin (5-hydroxytryptamine or 5HT) – one of the chemicals found in the brain which can influence the size of blood vessels throughout the body.

Further work by Professor Federigo Sicuteri in Florence,

and by Professor Lance and his colleagues in Australia, showed that the amount of serotonin present increased early in the attack and decreased in the later stages. Serotonin is contained in the platelets – the tiny disc-like bodies in the blood – and is released when the platelets come together. The platelets of people with migraine show an increased ability to clump together and to release serotonin during an attack.

Dr Edda Hanington of London has put forward the theory that an abnormality of platelet function is the primary disorder in migraine. Normally platelets clump together in response to a number of substances such as noradrenalin and adrenalin. As the platelets clump together they may block some tiny blood vessels in the brain and thus produce the warning symptoms.

Migraine and sleep research

Oddly enough some people find that if they sleep too long they may get a migraine. One American doctor reported improvement in his patients' migraine attacks when he reduced their sleeping time and lightened the depth of their sleep by having them repeatedly touched during the night. Some other people who get migraine during the night incorporate their dreams into the warning symptoms of the attack. Yet another group will get migraine if they go too long without sleep but most people who have a migraine attack feel better if they can go to sleep.

There are recurring cycles in the sleep pattern which appear to be regulated by the nervous system. One such cycle is characterized by rapid eye movement (REM). This period of REM sleep is associated with dreaming as well as an increase in heart rate, respiration and blood flow. Professor E.D. Weitzman of New York has a special sleep laboratory in which continuous reading can be made of the subject's activity, whether he is awake or asleep. Professor Weitzman and Dr J.D. Dexter have shown that migraine headaches which occur at night could be linked with REM sleep and there is also good evidence that the chemical serotonin, which changes the size of blood vessels, is involved in the regulation of sleep cycles. REM sleep has been linked to an increase in the cerebral blood flow, and migraine may be associated with a stage of sleep when there are alterations in the cerebral blood flow and in circulating serotonin.

Testing new drugs

New drugs are constantly being made by chemists but if a pharmaceutical company wants to develop a new drug for migraine or any other purpose various tests have to be made before it can be used. Toxicity tests using laboratory animals must be done to see that it has no harmful effects, then the drug must be tested on people to see if it is effective and to find out the appropriate dose.

Trials on anti-migraine drugs are usually carried out on volunteers in migraine clinics or in units where a large number of patients with headaches are seen. Anyone participating in such a trial or test must be healthy and able to understand the meaning and purpose of the trial. Usually they have to be aged between eighteen and sixty, have at least two but not more than eight headaches a month, and most important, they must not be taking any pills which might interfere with the action of the drug that is being tested.

To start with 'open' trials are done. Both the patient and the doctor know what drug is being taken and the patient is asked to comment on its effectiveness and whether there are any side-effects. Once some idea of the suitable dose has been found, a 'double blind' trial is done. In this type of trial both active and inactive (placebo) pills are given and neither the doctor nor the patient knows which is which. This is done so that any comments on the effectiveness of the medicine will not be prejudiced either in favour or against the drug that is being given. It is very common for people to feel better when they are given a new pill, particularly if they know that their doctor is interested in them and in the action of the pills. This improvement, known as the placebo-reaction, may be as high as 30 per cent.

Testing a new drug is a very complicated and expensive process and may cost the drug company a great deal of money and take three or four years to complete.

Migraine clinics

What you should know about clinics
Throughout the world there are now a number of clinics dealing specially with migraine and other types of headache. These

clinics differ slightly in their approach and organization from country to country. Throughout this book I have referred to the findings at the migraine clinic where I work in London. In this clinic and others like it, people with migraine are able to see doctors specializing in migraine. They can have their investigations and examinations carried out by specialists and receive the appropriate treatment.

Whatever the difference in the running of migraine clinics in Western countries, whether they are funded by the state or by charging the patients, there is general agreement about the treatment. Today most doctors believe that a great deal can be done in specialist migraine centres in the way of diagnosis, treatment and research.

To attend a migraine clinic in many countries such as Britain and Australia it is usually necessary for you to be referred first by your family doctor. He will give you a letter or make an appointment for you at the nearest one. Most migraine clinics are located in hospitals, but if there is no suitable clinic nearby the doctor may send you to the neurological department or the general medical out-patients department of your nearest hospital.

Apart from the hospital clinics there are a small number of specialist clinics which are run independently of hospitals and are devoted exclusively to migraine and headache. The great advantage of these specialist clinics is that people can be seen when they are actually having an attack.

The City of London Migraine Clinic

One of the first migraine clinics to see people during an acute attack was the City Migraine Clinic, now the City of London Migraine Clinic, which I helped establish. It was opened in 1970 and provides a centre for the treatment of and research into migraine. Patients are either referred by their general practitioner or come for emergency treatment in an attack. In the years that it has been in existence over four thousand patients have been seen during an acute attack.

Some of the questions I have been asked most frequently during the ten years I have been associated with the Clinic are worth including here.

Why do we need migraine clinics? People like to go somewhere where there is expertise and where their condition is taken seriously. If you have a headache you do not want to be told that it is 'just a headache' and sent away after a few minutes. In a migraine clinic you will be treated by doctors who have a specialized interest in migraine and other kinds of headache as well as an up-to-date knowledge of the best methods of treatment.

The specialized migraine clinic is in the unique position of being able to see people coming in with a severe headache almost immediately. They can be taken to a quiet room and have a history taken and an examination done by the doctor. Anyone who has been to the casualty department of a busy hospital will know that the waiting time there can be very long, even an hour or more. In the specialist clinic as soon as the patient comes in he is seen by the doctor, given the appropriate treatment and then allowed to lie down and go to sleep if he wishes.

Furthermore, migraine clinics give the doctors an opportunity of seeing patients during an attack and carrying out research into what happens during this vital time.

Is a migraine clinic primarily for research?   Clinics are very important in migraine research because relatively little is known about what happens in a migraine attack. If patients are not seen at this time it is very difficult to obtain information about the kind of biochemical and other changes which occur during an attack. Between attacks people with migraine are to all intents and purposes normal.

However, even though research may be one of the principal concerns of the clinic, you come first. The clinics are there to see and treat you and no research can be done without your willing and active co-operation.

Who runs a migraine clinic?   Although the main symptom of migraine is headache, there is no doubt that a great number of people also have other symptoms. About 90 per cent are nauseated, 50 per cent vomit at some time and 20 per cent have diarrhoea as well, and some people also have difficulty in passing water. During an attack it is not unusual to feel cold and shivery or, conversely, flushed and hot. Because of the general nature of the symptoms and changes which occur in an attack, many people think that a general physician should be the one involved in the care of a migraine sufferer. Indeed, most people with migraine are seen and treated by their family doctor and do not need to go to clinics. However, clinics run by specialists do, of course, provide a specialized service.

Many clinics, for instance, are run by neurologists. These are doctors who are skilled in the diagnosis and treatment of disorders of the nervous system. They are arguably most likely to be able to make a differential diagnosis between migraine and other types of headache.

At least one successful migraine clinic in the United States is run by an ear, nose and throat surgeon; many eye specialists have a particular interest in migraine too.

One thing, however, is certain, and that is that those who do run migraine clinics are all really interested in migraine and the patients who come to them.

Who should go to a migraine clinic? Sometimes it is the person with migraine who decides that he wants to go and see a specialist, perhaps because for one reason or another the treatment that he has had so far has not helped him as much as he thinks it should have. In most cases, however, it is the family doctor who decides that further help should be sought, particularly if there is some doubt as to whether the symptoms are caused by migraine.

Where are the migraine clinics? Most migraine clinics are in the out-patient departments of a general hospital and are open on one or two days a week. The advantage of having a migraine clinic in a large hospital is that there is a back-up staff to provide any investigatory services which may be necessary, such as X-rays, computerized axial tomography (CAT scan, see page 56), electroencephalograms, and so on. Patients with different types of headache can be diagnosed and treated, and if there are any neurosurgical emergencies, a neurosurgeon is on hand.

The disadvantage is that hospital clinics are usually held only once or twice a week and very few of them are prepared to give specialist help to those who come with an acute attack.

Small clinics devoted to migraine are able to give a more personal service. You are more likely to see the same doctor on each visit and the waiting time will probably be very much less. You would also know that any doctor working there has a particular interest in migraine.

In practice, both types of clinic offer a valuable service: those in a large hospital can provide all the necessary special facilities and smaller clinics can see people quickly and give emergency treatment to anyone who comes in during an acute attack.

A list of the hospitals or clinics which have a special interest in migraine is given on page 104.

What will I get from my clinic? From earliest times human beings have been concerned with pain and how to get rid of it. Headache is one of the commonest forms of pain and one of the things you will probably want from your headache clinic is relief of this pain. However, total relief of head pain is relatively rare. What the clinics can offer is a lessening of the pain, an explanation of the mechanism which triggered it off, and an assurance that in the great majority of cases there is no serious underlying cause.

If there is something you do not understand about your headache or its treatment, ask for an explanation at the clinic. The doctors are there primarily to help you. It is important that the nature of the treatment should be understood and that all medicines are taken as prescribed. I have known cases where a person undergoing what was supposed to be preventive treatment used only to take a tablet *during* an attack. Some people even take pain-killers two or three times a day when they are pain-free.

Can I be treated without drugs? There are now several migraine clinics where special emphasis is put on one particular type of treatment, such as biofeedback or acupuncture. If you want to try to beat your headaches without drugs you may want to ask your doctor about these special clinics.

An alternative approach to reducing or preventing headaches without the use of drugs is one you can learn for yourself and practise at home without attending a clinic. Stress, as I have mentioned throughout this book, is often a major contributory factor to both migraine and tension headaches, and many people find that learning to relax is a great help. To make this book complete, therefore, a special chapter on this important subject has been added here by Jane Madders, who is a leading authority on the treatment of stress and teaches relaxation at migraine classes.

12   STRESS AND RELAXATION

by Jane Madders, Dip P Ed, MCSP

Stress can be the spice of life. No one can live without some stress and tension, and when it is well managed it becomes the spur to action, a stimulus which enables us to adapt to changing situations and to meet the challenges of life. Managed badly it has become one of the killers in the modern world as well as causing much illness and inefficiency at work, and disrupting personal relationships.

Most people who have migraine or tension headaches will be well aware that physical fatigue and emotional states such as excitement, anger, frustration, prolonged spells of alertness and arousal can trigger their attacks. Stress may not necessarily be the root cause but can be the major precipitating factor.

There is a close relationship between muscle tension and emotional states and there is now plenty of evidence to show that various techniques of relaxation can help to induce a state of calm. It is worth remembering that it is not so much the stressful situation that causes the trouble but our reaction to it, and this we can learn to modify.

For more than thirty years I have taught relaxation to patients suffering from tension headaches and migraine. I worked in close collaboration with Dr M. Hay, the consultant at the Birmingham Migraine Clinic in England who has done much to add to our understanding of migraine. Most of the men and women attending the classes came because they themselves recognized that stress and fatigue tension played a big part in their attacks so they were well motivated to learn how to relax. When we checked them later we found that most had received considerable benefit from applying relaxation techniques to their daily living situations. Their attacks had become less frequent, were less intense and did not last as long as before. They reported other benefits also. Some were delighted to discover that they could manage long journeys without getting a migraine, and vacations which had once been a nightmare became a pleasure; sleep was often better and many were taking fewer or no drugs.

As a one-time migraine sufferer myself, I know that these techniques may not provide total cure. Although I have had no migraine or severe headaches for over twenty years I know that it would only require a prolonged period of extra stress coupled with dietary indiscretions to rouse the sleeping monster. So I take my own medicine which is relaxation, and it really is effective. It is a self-help method which involves no drugs, is safe and well worth using for its added benefits.

There is of course much more to relaxation than lying down and going limp. The first priority is to understand more about tension headaches and migraine. This removes some of the lonely fear that is common, and which this book will help to dispel.

Then it is important to understand a little about the effects of stress on the body and why relaxation helps. Many people have doubts at first and cannot see how relaxing arms and legs can possibly help a headache. This healthy scepticism is a good start because to be really effective relaxation techniques must be based upon the kind of conviction that comes from understanding and experience.

What is stress?

As individuals we are unique, unprecedented and unrepeatable, the result of the interplay between our inherited characteristics, early childhood experiences and the kind of battering that life has given us since. So what one person regards as stressful may be sheer pleasure for another. Some seem to need all the excitement they can get, work best under pressure, emerge unruffled from a heated argument or a telling off by someone in authority, and enjoy conflict. Others feel things more acutely, are profoundly moved by emotional experiences, take criticism very much to heart and may be exhausted by their feelings. These very qualities make them invaluable people, provided they can manage their stress reactions, because they may be more tuned in to other people and are more aware of their feelings and needs. These are the people who gain very much from learning to relax. So try to recognize the type of situations that make you tense, and identify the source of your stresses. These may, for example, be people, pressures at work, changes in routine (moving jobs, changing house, vacations) noise or lack of sleep. Then learn to react to them in a more relaxed way.

What happens in stress?

Hans Selye, the Austrian born endocrinologist, when working at the University of Montreal, defined stress as the general response of the body to any demand, pleasant or unpleasant made upon it. It is the rate of wear and tear on the body. This response has survival value and is intended to prepare the body for vigorous physical action when life is threatened. The first thing that happens when we recognize danger (whether it is real or imaginary) is that our muscles immediately tense for action, and we may make a gasp in breathing. (Remember this when we consider how the opposite condition, muscle relaxation and calm breathing, can help in calming down.) Then the message is received by the brain and biochemicals are poured into the bloodstream and nervous messages are passed to all parts of the body to prepare it to fight or to escape. A host of physical and chemical changes occur. It may be that migraine sufferers are particularly vulnerable to the action of catecholamines, the hormones released by the adrenal glands in stress.

Then, when the danger is over and the biochemicals used up in action, the body settles down to normal and no harm is done. However, if these changes are maintained for long periods unnecessarily this may lead to a variety of physical and mental disorders.

We react in the same way to frustration at work, anger when we are driving, domestic problems, or excitement at new situations. But stress reactions that were appropriate for our primitive ancestors are no longer suited to the stresses of modern civilization.

A certain amount of tension is necessary for success, and up to a point, the more aroused you are, the better you cope. But only up to a point. There is a stage of mental and physical fatigue at which the normal healthy person will take steps to recover by rest, relaxation or a change of occupation. Many people, however, especially those prone to headaches, feel they must drive themselves beyond this point towards exhaustion. They take on more and more tasks and seem almost afraid to let up. Indeed, if they have got to this point, stopping their activity may trigger off a migraine.

So try to assess how much stress you can tolerate, have the

courage to say 'no' sometimes and use relaxation techniques to renew your energy. You will work all the better for this and will later be able to take more stress in your stride.

Learning how to relax

Muscle relaxation, which can be learnt as a physical skill and then applied to daily situations, is a simple technique that can be mastered by almost anyone. It will relieve unnecessary muscle tension and the aches and pains that this brings (especially in the muscles at the back of the neck and shoulders, the forehead and scalp); it can help you cope with stress; it can raise your threshold of pain tolerance; and some migraine sufferers find that they can markedly reduce the actual pain of an attack by relaxing through it.

Although we are continually being reminded of the ill effects of excessive tension and may be well aware of it in ourselves, we are rarely shown just how to relax. The following exercises are an introduction to ways of recognizing tension. You can get further information from my book published in this series, called *Stress and Relaxation*, or by attending classes.

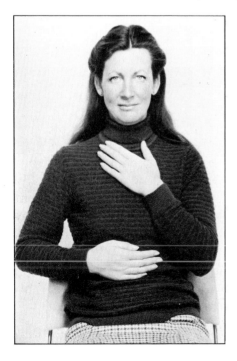

Breathing

Anxious panic breathing is in the upper part of the chest. If you are overbreathing as a habit you may be getting rid of too much carbon dioxide and causing an inbalance of chemicals in the blood. This can give rise to many unpleasant sensations — more anxiety, headaches, feeling faint, tingling of the hands. So check up on your breathing this way.

Put one hand on the top of your chest and the other over the navel. As you breathe in, your lower hand should rise and the top one hardly at all.

Breathe in gently, then breathe out slowly taking a little longer than the in breath. Pause for a moment then continue breathing calmly and evenly emphasising the slower outbreath.

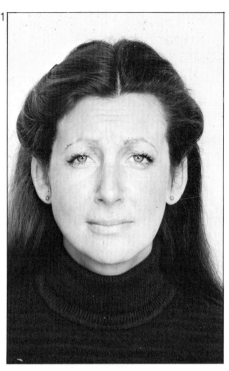

Recognizing tension

1. Tense forehead muscles can cause headaches and vice versa. Let these muscles relax so that your forehead feels a little wider and higher than before.

2. Clench your teeth and feel the ridge of muscle it produces at your temples. If you often grit your teeth during the day (or even at night) it may trigger off a headache.

3. Many people are unaware how tightly they hold their shoulders all day. Hunch them up towards your ears just the amount you do when you are anxious (3). Recognize this and then let them drop. Notice tension in your shoulders during your everyday occupations and, if you have been sitting still for long periods, wriggle your shoulders about.

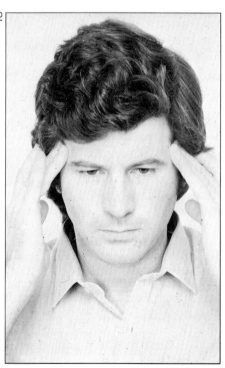

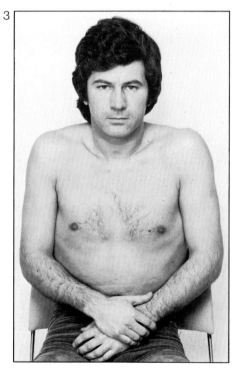

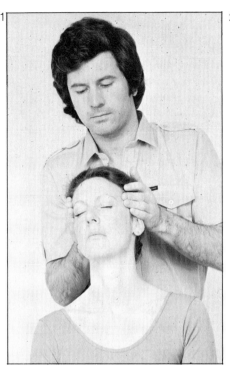

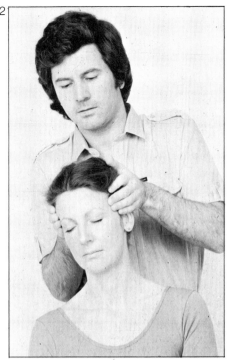

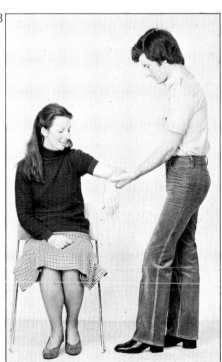

Testing relaxation with a partner

1 and 2. Your partner can help you to relax your neck muscles. He stands behind you and holds your head, placing it into a good position: upright and neither bent sideways nor thrust forward. The partner moves your head very gently and slightly (1 and 2) and if your neck muscles are relaxed he will be able to do this without hindrance, finishing with your head back in the middle.

3. Your partner places one hand under your elbow and the other under your wrist. Without you helping or hindering him he lifts it and moves it gently. He will be able to tell you if you have relaxed and whether your arm feels loose and heavy.

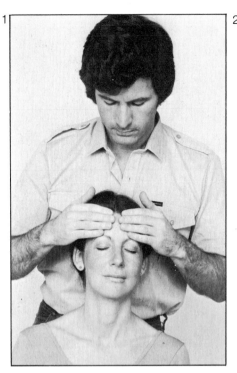

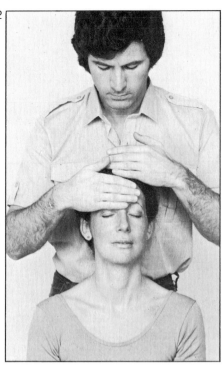

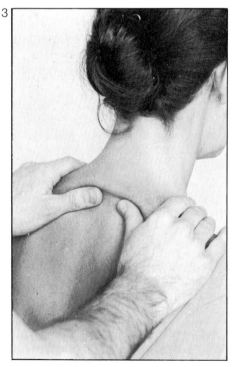

Massage

1 and 2. Massage helps muscles to relax and gives a general feeling of pleasant tranquillity. Your head should rest against your partner. Close your eyes, while he very gently smoothes his fingers sideways along your forehead to the temples (1). After a while he can change to relaxed smoothing upwards, one hand after the other (2).

3. The skin is rolled firmly, but not uncomfortably, upwards. After a while the shoulders feel a warm glow and are more relaxed.

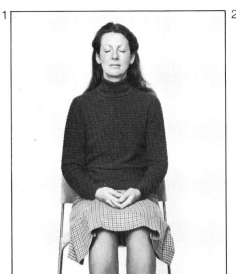
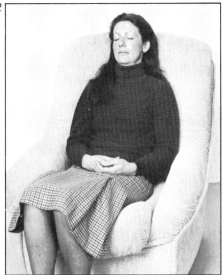

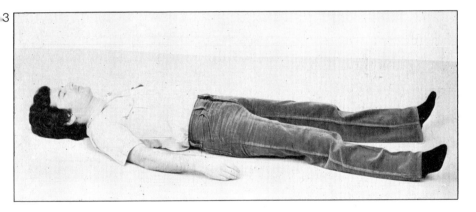

'Time-out' relaxation

You can get much help from snatching brief spells of relaxation (even three minutes will be valuable) sitting in an upright chair (1). You can do this anywhere – in a bus, in the office – whenever you are short of time but want to simmer down. Use an armchair if you can (2). Deeper relaxation may be obtained by lying flat on a firm surface (3). Choose the position that suits you best.

Biofeedback

Biofeedback instruments are useful because they show you when you are relaxed, and what it was you did to manage it. I have used them in my classes for the past seven years but only as an extra aid to the relaxation training.

The instrument we have found most helpful is the one that measures general arousal in the autonomic (involuntary) nervous system by measuring the changes in the electrical resistance of the skin. Such changes occur continually in everyday life without our noticing them. Instruments like the Relaxometer translate them into an audible signal. Changes in the pitch of the signal make you immediately aware when your arousal level has changed. You can use this knowledge to learn to relax at will, first of all in calm surroundings and later in more stressful situations.

"Stop" — a quick relaxation technique

You will find this quick and simple technique surprisingly effective in an emergency. You can use it when you are frustrated and angry, or anxious before interviews, social occasions, or at any time when you want to calm down quickly. An advantage is that no one will notice what you are doing.

When you realise that you are getting tense say sharply to yourself "STOP" (i.e. "stop fussing"). As you do this you are breathing out. Take a breath in, then breathe out SLOWLY, and as you do so, let your shoulders drop and relax your hands. Pause for a moment.

Take another breath in and this time as you breathe out relax your forehead and your jaw (because many people frown and grit their teeth when they are frustrated or anxious).

Pause for a moment then as you breathe calmly again become aware of the quietening down sensation. Then say to yourself: "I feel calmer. I feel relaxed."

This is worth practising. It can be a great help.

There are many different ways of learning to relax. Some people like the mechanical help of biofeedback, others prefer the simplicity of muscle relaxation, or the mysticism of some forms of meditation. It is up to each of us to find the method best suited to ourselves for controlling our responses to stress and thus our migraine and headaches.

13 CONCLUSION

Headaches and migraine bring misery to millions every year. It is therefore very important that people who suffer from them should know as much as possible about ways to avoid or to treat the pain, and I hope that this book will have provided all the up-to-date information and practical guidance you need. Everyone's problems will be different and it will of course be up to you to find the method of coping that best suits your own particular case. I hope at least that knowing what might be causing your discomfort and what kind of help might be available to you will ensure that you find the best possible way to deal with the problem.

If you need further information some of the organizations listed overleaf, which specialize in migraine, should be able to help with your enquiries.

USEFUL ADDRESSES

NATIONAL ORGANIZATIONS

UNITED STATES
American Pain Society
340 Kingsland Street
Nutley, NJ 07110

National Migraine Association
5252 North Western Avenue
Chicago, IL 60625

BRITAIN
British Migraine Association
178A High Road
Byfleet
Weybridge
Surrey KT14 7ED

The Migraine Trust
45 Great Ormond Street
London WC1

CANADA
The Migraine Foundation
390 Brunswick
Toronto
Ontario

SPECIALIST CLINICS
(arranged alphabetically by city or town within each country – for a complete list contact your national migraine organization or department of health)
British, Irish and Australasian readers must obtain a covering letter from their doctor before requesting an appointment for consultation.

UNITED STATES
Michigan Headache & Neurological Institute
3120 Professional Drive
Ann Arbor, MI 48104
(Attn: Joel Saper, MD)

Beverly Hills Headache & Pain Medical Group
9400 Brighton Way (Suite 410)
Beverly Hills, CA 90210
(Attn: Gunnar Heuser, MD, PhD)

Diamond Headache Clinic Ltd
5252 North Western Avenue
Chicago, IL 60625
(Attn: Seymour Diamond, MD)

The New England Center for Headache
40 East Putnam Avenue
Cos Cob, CT 06807
(Attn: Alan M. Rapoport, MD)

Houston Headache Clinic
1213 Hermann Drive
Houston, TX 77004
(Attn: Ninan T. Mathew, MD)

The Headache Research Foundation
Patient Care Division
Professional Office Suite at Faulkner Hospital
(Suite 5975)
Jamaica Plain, MA 02130
(Attn: Mrs Liz Heatley)

Montefiore Hospital Headache Unit
111 East 210th Street
Bronx, NY 10467

Ryan Headache Center
Mercy Doctors Building (Suite 537)
621 South New Ballas Road
St Louis, MO 63141
(Attn: Robert E. Ryan Sr, MD)

Headache Group of the Southwest
1402 North Miller Road (Suite F-5)
Scottsdale, AZ 85257
(Attn: G. Scott Tyler, MD)

CANADA
Sunnybrook Medical Center
Room 4300 – B4
2075 Bayview Avenue
Toronto
Ontario M4N 3M5
(Attn: John Edmeads, MD)

1030 West Georgia Street
Vancouver
B.C. V6E 2Y6
(Attn: Samuel E. C. Turvey, MD)

BRITAIN

All correspondence should be addressed to:
The Secretary, The Migraine Clinic

Birmingham and Midland Eye Hospital
Church Street
Birmingham B3 2NS

Department of Neurology
Addenbrooke's Hospital
Cambridge CB2 1QE

Neurological Unit
Northern General Hospital
Ferry Road
Edinburgh EH5 2DQ

Department of Neurology
Royal Devon & Exeter Hospital
(Wonford)
Barrack Road
Exeter EX2 5DW

Southern General Hospital
1345 Govan Road
Glasgow G51 4TF

Hull Royal Infirmary
Anlaby Road
Hull HU3 2JZ

City of London Migraine Clinic
22 Charterhouse Square
London EC1

Princess Margaret Clinic
Charing Cross Hospital
Fulham Palace Road
London W6 8RF

Regional Neurological Centre
Newcastle General Hospital
Newcastle-upon-Tyne NE4 6BE

Radcliffe Infirmary
Woodstock Road
Oxford OX2 6HE

IRELAND

People suffering severe migraine might be referred to the Neurological Clinic of one the following hospitals:

Cork Regional Hospital
Wilton
Cork

Limerick Regional Hospital
Dooradoyle
Co. Limerick

Adelaide Hospital
Peter Street
Dublin 8

St Vincent's Hospital
Elm Park
Dublin 4

The Regional Hospital
Galway

AUSTRALIA
Neurology Clinic
Flinders Medical Centre
South Road
Bedford Park, SA 5042

Headache Clinic
Royal Brisbane Hospital
Herston Road
Herston, QLD 4006

Neurology Clinic
Prince Henry Hospital
Anzac Parade
Little Bay, NSW 2036

Pain Management Centre
520 Collins Street
Melbourne, VIC 3000

Pain Clinic
Sir Charles Gairdner Hospital
Verdun Street
Nedlands, WA 6009

Neurological Department
Royal North Shore Hospital
Pacific Highway
St Leonards, NSW 2065

Headache and Pain Clinic
Queen Elizabeth Hospital
Woodville Road
Woodville, SA 5011

NEW ZEALAND
Neurological Clinic
Auckland Hospital
Park Road
Grafton
Auckland

Clinical School of Medicine
Christchurch Hospital
Riccarton Avenue
Christchurch

Wellington Clinical School
Wellington Hospital
Riddiford Street
Wellington

ACKNOWLEDGEMENTS

My thanks are due to my secretary, Mrs P. Kasserer, without whose assistance and encouragement this book would never have been written; and to Diana Davies and Piers Murray Hill for their helpful and sympathetic editing.

The material for this book is based on the information that my patients have given me and I am grateful to them and my colleagues at the City of London Migraine Clinic for their help. I would also like to express my gratitude to my many colleagues throughout the world who share my interest in migraine and from whose work I have quoted extensively. In particular I would like to thank John Graham and Mervyn Eadie for writing forewords to the American and Australian editions respectively.

The case histories in the book are based on my clinical experience but neither they nor the names relate to any particular individual.

The chapter on Stress and Relaxation has been written by Jane Madders and I am most grateful to her for this.

Finally I would like to thank Martin Dunitz for his advice and help.

Marcia Wilkinson, London 1981

The publishers are grateful to the following for permission to reproduce photographs: John Clutterbuck, New South Wales (page 79); Ed Cooper, California (page 51); Bill Ling, London (pages 24, 32-3, 67, 97-101); Miller Services, Toronto (pages 47, 71, 78); Adrian Pope, London (pages 11, 28, 65); and Doug Wilson, Washington (pages 37, 54, 83).

The diagrams on pages 16 and 61 were drawn by Barbara Leaning. The studio modelling was done by Evelyn Duval and John Weller, and the furniture was kindly lent by William Whitely Ltd, Bayswater, London. Finally thanks are due to Jennifer Eaton, BSc, MSc, MPS, for information on British, North American and Australian drug name equivalents.

INDEX

abdominal migraine, 80–1
acetaminophen, 50, 57–8, 68
acupuncture, 63, 93
adrenalin, 11, 87, 88
alcohol, 31, 34–5, 68, 69
allergies, food, 32–4, 49
altitude headaches, 72
amines, 32, 34, 35
analgesic abuse headache, 60
anticonvulsants, 62
anti-depressant drugs, 63
anti-sickness drugs, 57, 80
aspirin, 23, 50, 57–8, 68
aura, 7, 19–20

benzodiazepines, 58
beta-blockers, 63
biofeedback, 53, 67, 93, 101–2
blood pressure, raised, 9, 75
blood vessels, 10–11, 68, 86–8
brain tumours, 73, 84

Calpol, 50, 80, 81
CAT scan, 26, 56, 73
catecholamines, 11, 87, 96
cerebral angiography, 87
cheese, trigger factors, 31–2
children and migraine, 15–16, 29, 49, 72, 78–84
'Chinese restaurant' syndrome, 69–70
chocolate, 31, 34
classical migraine, 7, 9, 19–20, 35
clonidine, 63
cluster headaches, 8, 9, 35, 60, 63, 69, 74
codeine, 68
coffee, 31, 33, 58
compresses, hot and cold, 52

contraceptive pills, 43

daily headaches, 9, 60
depression, 63, 68
diarrhoea, 23–4, 91
diazepam, 62
diuretics, 25
dopamine, 11, 32, 87
drugs, 23, 57–60, 62–3, 89

effort migraine, 36–7
electroencephalogram, 56, 62
emotional stress, 35, 48
encephalitis, 73, 84
ergotamine tartrate, 58–60, 63
excitement, trigger factor, 29, 79
exercise, trigger factor, 36–8
explorers' headache, 71–2
eyes, blood vessels, 86; infections, 10; ophthalmoplegic migraine, 26; visual disturbances, 7, 19–21, 22, 37–8, 80

fever, 25, 73
5HT antagonists, 60, 62–3
food, trigger factors, 30–5, 49, 69–70

giddiness, 22

hangovers, 69
head injuries, 75–7
hearing difficulties, 22
heartbeat, rapid, 25
hemianopia, 19–20
hemiplegic migraine, 25–6
histamine, 12, 35
hormones, 11, 41–4, 87, 96
'hot-dog' headaches, 70
hunger, trigger factor, 48–9
hypoperfusion, 86

'ice-cream' headache, 70
inheritance of migraine, 17–18
intelligence and migraine, 14–15, 81

light, trigger factors, 29–30, 49, 64, 65
lithium, 63

malaliquid bite, 10
massage, 52, 67
Medihaler, 50
meditation, 53, 67, 102
meningitis, 73, 84
menopause, 15, 43–4
menstruation, 9, 15, 41–2
methysergide, 62–3
metoclopramide, 23, 40, 57, 80
migraine, areas of pain, 22; clinics, 12, 89–93; diagnosis, 9–10; duration, 9; research, 85–93; sufferers, 13–18; symptoms, 10–12, 19–26; treatment, 22, 48–55, 56–63; trigger factors, 27–40; types of, 7–8
'migraine equivalent', 26
monosodium glutamate, 69–70
mountain sickness, 72

nasal stuffiness, 8, 25
nausea, 7, 8, 23–4, 57, 91
neck, 10, 77
nicotinic acid, 68
noise, trigger factor, 29–30, 54–5, 64
noradrenalin, 11, 87, 88
numbness, 21

octopamine, 32
oestrogen, 41–2, 43–4
Olesen, Prof J, 86
ophthalmoplegic migraine, 26

pain, 22–3, 64–5, 68, 97
pain-killers, 50, 52, 57–8, 68, 80
paracetamol, 50, 57–8, 68, 78
peridone, 57
pizotifen, 62–3
platelets, 17, 88
pregnancy, 9, 15, 42–3
progesterone, 41–2, 43–4

propranolol, 63
prostaglandins, 12
psychological factors, 67–8

relaxation, 52–3, 67, 93, 94–102
Reyes disease, 50

scalp tenderness, 24
sedatives, 58, 62
serotonin, 12, 39, 87–8
sexual intercourse, 72
Sicuteri, Prof F, 87
sinusitis, 73, 74–5
sleep, 28–9, 50–2, 58, 61, 88
smells, trigger factors, 39–40
speech disturbances, 21
spinal injuries, 77
stomach upsets, 23–4, 80
'Stop' technique, 102
stress, 11, 29, 35–6, 48, 58, 87, 93, 94–7
strokes, 73
sumatriptan, 60

teeth, dental problems, 10
temperature, extremes of, 49–50
tempero-mandivular joint, 10
temporal arteritis, 73, 74
tension headaches, 9, 60, 61, 64–8, 82, 94–5
thermography, 86
tingling sensations, 21
tranquillizers, 62
travel sickness, 18, 81–2
trigeminal neuralgia, 74
trigger factors, 27–40
tyramine, 31–2, 33, 35

ultrasonography, 86–7
urination, frequency, 24, 25, 91

visual disturbances, 7, 19–21, 22, 37–8, 80
vitamin A, 71–2
vomiting, 23–4, 91

water retention, 25, 42
weather, trigger factors, 38–9, 50
weekend headache, 27–8
women and migraine, 9, 15, 41–7

yoga, 53, 67

All Optima books are available at your bookshop or newsagent, or can be ordered from the following address:

Optima, Cash Sales Department,
PO Box 11, Falmouth, Cornwall TR10 9EN

Please send cheque or postal order (no currency), and allow 60p for postage and packing for the first book, plus 25p for the second book and 15p for each additional book ordered up to a maximum charge of £1.90 in the UK.

Customers in Eire and BFPO please allow 60p for the first book, 25p for the second book plus 15p per copy for the next 7 books, thereafter 9p per book.

Overseas customers please allow £1.25 for postage and packing for the first book and 28p per copy for each additional book.